PRACTICAL FORENSIC PATHOLOGY

PRACTICAL FORENSIC PATHOLOGY

Charles V. Wetli, M.D.

Deputy Chief Medical Examiner
Dade County Medical Examiner Department
Dade County, Florida

Clinical Associate Professor of Pathology
Department of Pathology
University of Miami—School of Medicine
Miami, Florida

Roger E. Mittleman, M.D.

Associate Medical Examiner
Dade County Medical Examiner Department
Dade County, Florida

Clinical Associate Professor of Pathology
Department of Pathology
University of Miami—School of Medicine
Miami, Florida

Valerie J. Rao, M.D.

Associate Medical Examiner
Dade County Medical Examiner Department
Dade County, Florida

Clinical Assistant Professor of Pathology
Department of Pathology
University of Miami—School of Medicine
Miami, Florida

IGAKU-SHOIN 1944

IGAKU-SHOIN New York • Tokyo

Cover Design by M 'N O Production Services, Inc.
Typesetting by The Clarinda Company
Printing and Binding by Arcata Graphics/Halliday

Published and distributed by
IGAKU-SHOIN Medical Publishers, Inc.
1140 Avenue of the Americas, New York, N.Y. 10036

IGAKU-SHOIN Ltd.,
5-24-3 Hongo, Bunkyo-ku, Tokyo

Library of Congress Cataloging-in-Publication Data

Wetli, Charles V.
Practical forensic pathology.

Includes index.
1. Autopsy. 2. Forensic pathology. I. Mittleman, Roger E. II. Rao, Valerie J. III. Title. [DNLM: 1. Autopsy—methods. 2. Forensic Medicine—methods. 3. Pathology—methods. W 825 W539p]
RA1063.4.W47 1988 614'.1 87-35275

ISBN: 0-89640-144-8 (New York)
ISBN: 4-260-14144-9 (Tokyo)

Printed and bound in USA

10 9 8 7 6 5 4 3 2 1

Foreword

Current residency training in anatomic pathology is primarily directed at the detection and identification of diseases and their effects, and the evaluation of current treatment modalities. Consequently, conceptual and technical aspects of the autopsy are directed toward organ systems, and the results are primarily for the benefit of the physician. Usually, very little training is afforded in the area of forensic pathology where disease processes may have nothing to do with the death of an individual, and where the autopsy findings are primarily of interest to nonmedical personnel. It is thus not surprising that the techniques and concepts that work well with the usual hospital autopsy are inapplicable to the forensic autopsy. Consequently, hospital-trained pathologists are often apprehensive and reluctant when called upon to perform an autopsy on an individual who apparently died in an unnatural mode. This is quite understandable, since the hospital-based pathologist is, in effect, being required to undertake a task for which he or she is inadequately trained.

Current texts on forensic pathology available to hospital pathologists primarily address the pathophysiology and pathologic changes induced by various injuries and the interpretation of injury patterns. They do not, however, address the practical issues of how to approach the autopsy of a trauma victim: what is important to describe, what measurements are needed, required procedures that are outside the scope of the hospital autopsy, and so forth. This book is an attempt to fill the gap between what is learned during a residency in Anatomic Pathology and the interpretation of the autopsy findings.

The procedures outlined in the text are to serve as guidelines to provide a practical approach to a case with medicolegal interest. The emphasis is on the documentation and preservation of evidence, not the interpretation of the findings. It is recognized that real circumstances may vary considerably from those where a well-established medical examiner system exists. Consequently, some procedures will be inapplicaable or impractical under some circumstances. Hopefully the reader will be able to utilize the concepts provided and apply them to the situation at hand. At the very least, we hope these guidelines will alleviate some of the anxiety experienced when the general pathologist is thrust into the world of medicolegal death investigation. It is hoped that this practical approach will enable the general hospital pathologist to adequately describe and document the essential features of a ''forensic case.'' In this way, crucial information is preserved. Problems with interpretation that go beyond the expertise of the pathologist can then be referred to specialists in the field.

Contents

PRACTICAL FORENSIC PATHOLOGY

CHAPTER 1

Concepts and Procedures for All Cases of Medicolegal Interest

INTRODUCTION

The responsibility for medicolegal death investigation varies according to political structure in different geographic locations. In a medical examiner system, the primary responsibility rests with the pathologist to determine the cause and manner of death and to interpret the autopsy findings. In other circumstances, the responsible person may be a lay coroner or the commander of a military hospital, and the pathologist merely provides a report that is left to the interpretation of others. No matter what the circumstances, the autopsy should never be performed without as much information as possible concerning the scene of death, the terminal events, and the background of the victim. It is to be emphasized that the autopsy is nothing more than a laboratory procedure where the results must be interpreted in the light of antecedent events. Conversely, knowledge of the death scene, terminal events, and background information modifies the approach to the autopsy. In the individual case, the circumstances of death determine what must be documented, measured, and tested.

When one compares the hospital autopsy to the forensic autopsy, it becomes apparent that significant differences necessitate modifying the approach to the autopsy and how the autopsy is to be reported. Initially, one of the most important differences is who gets autopsied and who authorizes the autopsy. In the hospital, the autopsy is authorized by the next of kin, usually at the request of a clinician. However, in medicolegal cases the type of case to be autopsied and the authorization are usually dictated by state law and/or local ordinance. Regardless of the law and local policy, it should be realized that the medicolegal autopsy has both a confirmatory and an evidentiary value, even when the cause of death appears obvious. The confirmatory aspect is best viewed as those findings which support the initial impression as to cause of death. By inference it also means that certain things were not found that would alter that initial impression. Thus, in a case where death appeared to be the result of a suicidal hanging, the autopsy would reveal the expected signs of such an asphyxial death. The fact that no other trauma was found would tend to negate a conjecture that the victim was first strangled and then made to appear like a victim of suicidal hanging. Evidentiary aspects of the autopsy therefore provide a record of the observations needed to confirm or refute a hypothesis of the terminal event. This evidence is in the form if diagrams, photographs, and the written report. Blood, tissue, or foreign objects recovered from the body and subsequently analyzed are also evidentiary and often require a documented chain of custody.

In the hospital setting, the case investigation is documented in the clinical record and the autopsy is the final laboratory procedure, which has primarily a correlative value. In the forensic case, the autopsy is often the initial laboratory procedure. The correlative aspects are subsequently developed in a variety of activities such as family conferences, legal proceedings, insurance adjustments, etc. The medicolegal autopsy is therefore but one of many investigative procedures that ultimately lead to a conclusion as to the cause, manner, and mechanism of death of a particular individual.

DEATH CERTIFICATION

Cause of Death

The cause of death may be simply defined as that disease or injury which resulted in the death of an individual. When there is a delay between the onset of a disease process or injury and the ultimate death of an individual, the proximate and the immediate causes of death must be distinguished. In essence, the immediate cause of death is that disease or injury which kills a person at a particular time and place. The proximate cause of death is the disease or injury which initiated a series of events that led directly to the immediate cause of death. This series of events must be a reasonable and foreseeable consequence of the initial event. Consider the example of a person who is stabbed in the abdomen during a fight and dies 2 weeks later in the hospital of peritonitis. The immediate cause of death is the peritonitis. Since this is a reasonable and foreseeable consequence of an abdominal wound of this nature, the proximate cause of death is therefore the stab wound of the abdomen. In this instance, the peritonitis is regarded as the dependent (i.e., on the stab wound) intervening factor, which, within a reasonable degree of medical probability, caused the death of that person at that time. The importance of this concept is that it allows one to form a conclusion as to the manner of death and, in this instance, allows for criminal prosecution of homicide. An independent supervening factor would be an event that would not be a reasonable and foreseeable consequence of the stab wound (e.g., a fall in the hospital resulting in fatal head injury). Sometimes the defense counsel in a criminal proceeding will argue that medical negligence is an independent supervening factor in death, and therefore the proximate event (stab wound) is not related to the immediate cause of death. Usually this is not a serious challenge, since it is recognized that nearly any medical procedure has an attendant risk. Even though a therapeutic error might have contributed to the death of the individual, this is usually not so pronounced as to negate the injury that put the person in the hospital in the first place.

When the injury results in virtually immediate death (e.g., gunshot wound to the head), the distinction between proximate and immediate causes of death does not apply—they are essentially the same thing.

For purposes of death certification, the length of time between the proximate and immediate causes of death is of no consequence. A man rendered paraplegic by a gunshot wound who dies 20 years later from pyelonephritis and a neurogenic bladder might still be classified as a homicide. However, because of statutes of limitation, the case may not be prosecutable.

Mechanism of Death

From a medical standpoint, the mechanism of death is th[illegible]logic derangement which is incompatible with life. Since most p[illegible]ined to think in terms of the mechanisms of disease processes, [illegible] find the mechanism of death confused with, or used in place o[illegible]th. Mechanisms of death have more than one possible etiolog[illegible]ect a pathophysiologic process that is a final common pathw[illegible]es, both natural and physical. Ventricular fibrillation, for exa[illegible]sm of death for both low-voltage electrocution and arterioscl[illegible]ry disease. Consequently, such terms (including "cardiac a[illegible]lly meaningless on a death certificate unless followed by an a[illegible]

Mechanism of death may also refer to the terminal p[illegible] an individual's life. In the case of a pedestrian struck by an [illegible] sequence of physical events leading to fatal injury is sometim[illegible] the kinematics or the mechanism of death. Whether the mechan[illegible]efers to pathophysiologic changes or to a sequence of physical [illegible]st be related back to the immediate and proximate cause of those e[illegible]

Manner of Death

At first glance, the manner of death appears quite simple: the death was natural, accidental, suicidal, or homicidal. However, this particular area has generated a great deal of discussion, confusion, and controversy regarding death certification. In part this is the result of undefined criteria, and the fact that certification of the manner of death is as much a function of tradition as it is of logic.

Although no uniform criteria exist for certifying the manner of death, the following discussion is offered as a guideline. Not all will agree with this discussion. However, it has proved to be a consistent, workable system over many years. For the novice it is intended to provide a starting place to develop a logical concept. For the more experienced, it will hopefully provide a forum for more discussion and the ultimate improvement of an admittedly imperfect system.

The autopsy is useful in determining the cause and mechanism of death, but by itself it virtually never determines the manner of death. This becomes fairly obvious when one considers that a contact gunshot wound of the head will look the same whether it is self-inflicted or the result of an execution. Likewise, sudden death resulting from severe coronary arteriosclerosis may in fact be a homicide if the terminal event occurred during an armed robbery or certain other felonies. The manner of death is thus an expressed opinion based upon all available knowledge of a particular case. This includes the autopsy findings, toxicologic results, scene of death, terminal events, and social and medical background information. Since the manner of death is based upon the sum total of information known up to a particular point in time, it may change upon the subsequent discovery of additional genuine information. Thus, the manner of death recorded on the death certificate is regarded as only "probable" and is based on a "preponderance of evidence." This is sometimes less than "certainty" or even "reasonable medical probability." In difficult cases, where background information may be quite sparse, the "preponderance of evidence" may only indicate a 51% preponderance as to the manner of death. And if there is no preponderance of evidence, the manner of death must remain unclassified until the proper information surfaces.

The major reason for expressing a manner of death is for statistical purposes. Should the criteria be too strict for a certain category, then an inordinate number of cases will remain unclassified. This is a detriment to families and to the society for which these statistics are useful for following trends. If, for example, an obvious suicide note is required in all instances where the manner of death is to be listed as suicide, then well over half such cases will remain unclassified. Since the manner of death expressed on a death certificate is for statistical purposes only, it should have no direct bearing on insurance contracts or criminal prosecution. For insurance purposes, contract law will determine the outcome of any settlement, which will be partially based on the particular manner of death. For criminal purposes, the law will also dictate a course of action. A manner of death correctly ascribed to homicide may be regarded, legally, as excusable, justifiable, first degree, etc. But these are legal definitions and proceedings properly beyond the scope of the forensic pathologist. Likewise, a manner of death listed as accidental does not preclude prosecution for manslaughter, should the circumstances be appropriate for that charge.

Death resulting from the progression of a disease process is regarded as "natural" only when there is no proximate or immediate environmental influence above what might be encountered in normal, everyday, or common experiences.

A fatal heart attack occuring during an altercation (viz a wordy quarrel without physical violence), while shoveling snow, or during sexual intercourse would be regarded as natural, since such events are common in everyday life.

Accidental deaths are those in which the person dies as the result of a hostile environment. Common examples are deaths from drowning, motor vehicle crashes, falls, etc. In the vast majority of cases, there is some form of human negligence involved, but this falls far short of suicidal or homicidal intent. Thus, alcoholic intoxication reduces a person's ability to function in an environment. The intoxication may lead to death in an automobile crash or by drowning at a beach party. Although negligent, the intoxication alone would not be sufficient to cause the manner of death to be classified as anything other than accidental. The alcoholic intoxication could, however, be properly listed as a contributory cause of death. Just as alcoholic intoxication can render a person susceptible to a relatively benign environment, so can natural disease. A fatal "heart attack" while swimming is usually regarded as an accidental death, with arteriosclerotic heart disease being a contributory factor. By convention, the decedent is "given the benefit of the doubt," since there would have been a possibility of survival had it not been for the environmental factor.

With automobile crash fatalities, there are two areas that are occasionally troublesome. The first is when the crash is thought to have been precipitated by a natural disease process, usually coronary arteriosclerosis. When there is little damage to the vehicle and only minor injuries to the driver, who has occlusive coronary arteriosclerosis, the manner of death is listed as natural. It is also listed as natural in those cases where there are severe injuries but also evidence that the heart had ceased to function prior to impact (e.g., a lacerated aorta with a minimal amount of internal bleeding). Should the injuries be severe and without evidence one way or the other to indicate the heart had ceased to function just prior to impact (e.g., basilar skull fracture, vehicular conflagration), then the manner of death is accidental.

The second area of controversy is those cases in which an intoxicated driver kills another person. Legally, the driver may be tried for manslaughter, and therefore some will argue that homicide should be listed on the death certificate. However, manslaughter is a legal term, and unless there is evidence of specific intent to kill a particular person with the vehicle (i.e., using an automobile as a weapon), we would describe the manner of death as accidental. In part this is from convention, but, more importantly, it provides a more logical statistical data base. Likewise, an intoxicated driver who crashes into a tree and dies would be regarded as an accidental death, not a suicide. The manner of death would, of course, change should there be evidence of intent to kill oneself or another person.

A death resulting from an acute and unintentional overdose of a drug or alcohol is regarded as an accidental death. A death from the medical complications resulting from chronic abuse of these substances, however, is generally classified as a natural death. This is based more on convention than on logic.

One could argue that since the medical complications are merely a mechanism of death in a drug or alcohol abuser, death from such complications should also be considered accidental. In that case, deaths from cigarette-induced lung cancer or asbestos-induced mesothelioma would also have to be considered accidental, since they have environmental etiologies. Since individuals who abuse substances such as alcohol, tobacco, or drugs are needlessly endangering their lives, one could also argue that the correct manner of death is suicide when death results from overdose or a medical complication. Finally, there is the argument that since alcoholism and drug addiction are diseases, both fatal overdoses and the medical complications of addiction should be regarded as natural deaths. Regardless of which philosophy is more pure or correct, the usual convention is to classify death from unintentional overdose as accidental and death from medical complications as natural.

Classifying a death as suicide not infrequently leads to discussions with the next of kin, who are unwilling to accept suicide as a manner of death. Usually this stems from a grief reaction marked by various aspects of denial. Less frequently, the protest is motivated by the rejection of an insurance claim with a suicide exclusionary clause. In either event, the preponderance of available evidence leading to a conclusion that the death was intentionally self-inflicted must be substantiated and explained. In most instances, suicide can be regarded as a first-degree self-murder. Background social and medical information and scene investigation are of primary importance in leading to a conclusion of suicide. The autopsy serves a confirmatory role in that it provides evidence that the decedent was not murdered and then the scene constructed to simulate a suicide.

A suicidal act occuring during a domestic quarrel, or while under the influence of drugs or alcohol, may usually be regarded as a second-degree self-murder, since the act was not previously planned (at least consciously). It may be argued that the emotional state of the decedent or the degree of intoxication was such that intent and culpability were severely diminished, and therefore the manner of death should be accidental or simply left unclassified. However, the acutely emotional or intoxicated state would have more likely lessened the inhibition of the person, thus making it easier to carry out the self-destructive act. Furthermore, it must be remembered that to kill oneself usually requires several deliberate steps (e.g., the gun must at least be obtained, positioned, and discharged). Consequently, the manner of death would be regarded as suicide.

"Russian roulette" is also regarded as a suicidal act. The rationale is that, first, the decedent was in control of the environment. Second, he or she took deliberate steps to prepare for the event (e.g., obtained the gun, unloaded it, placed one bullet in the chamber, closed the chamber, cocked the hammer, put the gun to the head, and pulled the trigger—a total of seven deliberate steps). Third, the chances of survival for the next moment were intentionally reduced from infinity to five out of six.

When death occurs as the result of the deliberate action of another, the manner of death (for the death certificate) is homicide. The key phrase is "deliberate action,'' and it must be distinguished from ''accidental,'' ''intentional,'' and ''unintentional.'' Intent is not a prerequisite for classifying a death as a homocide. Rather, intent is the purview of the courts, and the degree of intent will determine if the homicide is excusable or justifiable, or whether it is murder.

Frequently there is a temptation to equate ''unintentional'' with ''accidental,'' and this can lead to an erroneous classification of manner of death. Consider the situation of a hunter who shoots at a deer and misses, striking a companion instead. Although it is clear that the fatal shooting of the companion was not intentional, the shooting itself was, in fact, the deliberate action of another person. Consequently the correct manner of death is homicide, not accident. Similarly, if a person dies of a ruptured intracranial aneurysm during a barroom fist fight, the manner of death is homicide, even though there was no intent to seriously injure the other person. Cupability is the province of the courts and wil be determined by subsequent criminal and civil judicial proceedings.

In the majority of cases with sufficient information, the classification of manner of death is not problematical. Others will require a detailed and logical thought process and may still be controversial. The following scenario was once posed in the form of a question to a small group of experienced forensic pathologists:

> An elderly man, living at home, required continous oxygen administration because of endstage pulmonary disease. At his request, the wife disconnected the oxygen apparatus, and he died. The correct manner of death is:

1. Natural
2. Accident
3. Suicide
4. Homicide
5. Undetermined, pending inquest

Cogent arguments were made for virtually all of the choices and a consensus was not reached by the group. In our opinion, the correct answer is ''A''—the death was natural. The reason is that a person is always allowed to refuse medical treatment, even if it means that death is the inevitable consequence. In this case, the man simply elected to allow the natural progression of his disease process. The death would not be accidental, since the natural environment was, by itself, not hostile. The oxygen that sustained life was, in fact, an artificial environment which has certain dangers of its own. Since the man did nothing to hasten his own demise over that of natural progression, it is not suicide. Likewise, the wife did not hasten the natural progression of his disease by disconnecting the oxygen apparatus. She merely acquiesced in allowing her husband to survive or die in a natural environment. Hence, the death is not homicidal. The final choice is rejected, because a judicial inquiry, such as an inquest, is an inappropriate forum to determine the manner of death. (Obviously, coroners' systems, which frequently utilize the inquest to determine manner of death, will disagree with this!) Such a forum evaluates evidence in the light of law and therefore may appropriately address the question of criminal agency. However, the manner of death frequently has nothing to do with criminal agency, and death certification evolves from principles and a discipline independent of the law.

"Therapeutic Misadventure"

Deaths occuring during diagnostic or therapeutic procedures are occasionally difficult to certify as to manner of death. Generally, when death occurs during a high-risk procedure for the treatment of a potentially fatal disease, the death is regarded as natural. This includes operating room deaths for coronary artery disease, neurosurgical operations for brain tumors, etc. Also, the death is regarded as natural if the person succumbs to a known potential complication of a procedure—i.e., the calculated risk. Examples include excessive bleeding following a needle biopsy of the liver, anaphylactic reaction to radiation dye or a drug, or the complications of radiation therapy or chemotherapy. Such procedures are intended to benefit the patient, and yet each has a known calculated risk of complications that may prove fatal. However, when there is a complication that goes well beyond the calculated risk, then the death may be properly regarded as accidental. Examples include the inadvertent administration of the wrong drug, an excessive dose of a drug (e.g., 1 ml instead of 0.1 ml epinephrine), fatal hemolytic reaction because the wrong blood was given, the inadvertent injection of a chemical such as glutaraldehyde, or the administration of a drug known to be contraindicated. Such glaring errors are almost sure to lead to civil litigation for a wrongful death, and often there is at least the potential for criminal proceedings as well.

How the Incident Occurred

When the manner of death is something other than natural, a statement is generally required on the death certificate as to how the incident occurred. This is usually a simple remark, such as "Deceased shot self," "Deceased hit tree while driving automobile," or "Deceased was shot by other person(s)." On occasion this does become tricky, and the words should be chosen carefully. Situations demanding this attention are generally those deaths which occur during hospitalization (i.e., "therapeutic misadventures") or when the cause of death is a natural disease process but the manner of death is unnatural (e.g., murder by heart attack). Under such circumstances, one may then wish to modify the standard death certificate format by using words such as "associated with" instead of "due to." This is especially true when the exact mechanism or cause of death is not certain. Thus, the cause of death on the death certificate in a case of sudden unexpected death during anesthetic induction for a tonsillectomy might be worded as "ventricular fibrillation associated with induction of general anesthesia." How the incident occurred might be stated as "Deceased had cardiac arrhythmia during anesthesia induction." Likewise, a person who ruptures a berry aneurysm during a barroom brawl could have a death certificate worded as "rupture of berry aneurysm associated with emotional and physical stress." How the incident occurred could be stated as "Deceased had stroke during a fight."

The sole purpose for such wording on a death certificate is to avoid being definitive or dogmatic as to who or what may or may not be at fault. In the unexpected death during anesthesia induction, for example, it may eventually prove to be an arithmetic error or simply the unpredictable outcome of a cardiac conduction disturbance, with the role of anesthetic induction being speculative at best. Thus, when circumstances or mechanisms of death become complex or vague, the death certificate should be worded as simply and as broadly as possible. This allows for the eventual expression of a reasonable opinion as more information becomes available. It also avoids premature opinions that may prove indefensible in the future.

Scene Investigation

The primary reason for the pathologist (or his designee) to visit the death scene is to provide a correlative approach to the autopsy, which in turn will allow for a more meaningful interpretation of the autopsy findings. A secondary purpose is to provide information to the police to aid them in their initial phase of the investigation.

In this jurisdiction, pathologists frequently respond to death scenes. In other areas, reliance is made upon forensic investigators. When large distances are involved, the police may videotape the scene and send the videotape along with the body. In many areas, however, it is not possible or practical for the pathologist or a forensic investigator to visit the scene of death, and total reliance must therefore be made on the police report. The folllowing guidelines are offered to provide a protocol should you have the opportunity of responding to a death scene.

An expeditious response time will allow for a timely release of the body and enable the police to release the scene. Therefore, it is advisable to give the police your estimated arrival time so they can organize their activities. Remember that an expeditious response does not mean that traffic regulations are ignored! However, inordinate delay may have severe consequences—e.g., a fatality on the railroad tracks may back up trains for hundreds of miles if the response time is prolonged. The only truly essential items to bring with you are a camera and a pair of rubber gloves.

Upon arrival at the scene of death, you must first identify yourself and then locate the lead police investigator at the scene (this is not necessarily the detective in charge of the investigation). Ask where you may or may not walk, and what you may or may not touch. Next, request a summary of what is known about the incident, and request a guided tour of the scene. Photograph the body and the scene. Finally, with the police present, examine the body. Since you have on the rubber gloves, the police may request you empty the pockets of the deceased. Turn these items over to the police. When turning the body over, do so slowly and observe what lies beneath. In this way projectiles or other evidence may be revealed in relation to the original position of the body. If, while turning the body over, a gun is discovered (beneath the body or in the waistband of the pants), simply do not move until the police have taken their photographs and removed the gun.

As a matter of courtesy, notify the lead detective when you are leaving the scene. At that time it is appropriate to inquire as to whether any personnel of the police department or crime laboratory wish to be present during the autopsy. Whether or not a police representative attends, this helps to establish an avenue of communication for the mutually beneficial exchange of developing information.

Note that any opinions rendered at the scene are to be regarded as investigative and speculative. These initial opinions are never to be regarded as conclusive and, in fact, will change in major aspects in about half the cases as more information becomes available. It is therefore wise never to be dogmatic and always to remember that the purpose of your visit to the death scene is to allow a better correlation and interpretation of injuries with the environment of the death.

Finally, a summary of your observations at the scene should be recorded and included in the case file. Include the date and time you arrived at the scene, the name of the lead detective (or whoever you spoke with), a brief synopsis of the events as told to you by the police, your observations of the scene itself, your observations of the body, and your impression of the case at that point (e.g., multiple homicidal gunshot wounds). At the end, include a sentence which states that the foregoing information may be incomplete and speculative.

When to Autopsy

With every case referred to the medical examiner or coroner, the terminal event and circumstances under which the body was found, the medical history, and the scene of death must all be evaluated first. At this point one can formulate an idea as to the cause and manner of death, and determine what further investigation or procedures, including autopsy, are needed.

The determination as to whether to perform an autopsy, to do only an external examination, or simply to draw samples of blood for toxicologic testing will depend on a multitude of practical factors. Chief among these are the law, local policy, physical facility, personnel, and budgetary constraints. In some jurisdictions, an autopsy is done on all deaths suspected of being unnatural, as well as all apparently natural deaths where there is no medical history or where the death is not totally commensurate with the medical history. Others may simply externally examine and draw blood from "obvious" cases of suicide and from motor vehicle drivers, and only perform an external examination on apparent natural deaths where the decedent is above a certain age (for example, 50 years old). In our opinion, it is better to do an autopsy and obtain the necessary answers than to open the door to needless speculation and inquiry (which will take up much more time at a future date than an autopsy). In any event, the philosophical ideal will be tempered by practical realities. At the very least, however, an autopsy should be required in all suspected homicides, all cases where there is a possibility of criminal prosecution (e.g., hit-and-run victim), and all deaths in police custody. Autopsies should also be required for those cases where external evidence of trauma may be obscured or totally obliterated. These cases are usually those in advanced stages of decomposition (putrefaction, mummification, or adipocere formation) or those bodies removed from a conflagration where charring is extensive.

Objections to the Autopsy

The next of kin may object to an autopsy for personal or emotional reasons, because of social custom, or because of religious beliefs. The dilemma facing the pathologist is how to satisfy the statutory requirement while respecting the wishes, feelings, and beliefs of family members. To simply ignore the family will result in anger and resentment, which may eventually become manifest in legal action. The solution is to obtain a mutually agreeable compromise as to what procedure is to be done.

In our experience, personal objections often arise when there is a delay in the death (e.g., when a person dies after a week of hospitalization for injuries sustained in an automobile crash). Although the case may clearly come under the medical examiner/coroner jurisdiction, it would not be in anybody's best interest to proceed with an autopsy that will reveal nothing that has not already been substantially documented in the medical records. With a personal objection in this situation, an external examination and a review of the medical records will generally suffice, even if the precise terminal mechanism of death may not be clear (e.g., pulmonary thromboembolism, infection, etc.).

Personal objections to the autopsy may also stem from fears regarding mutilation of the body and/or defilement of the loved one. Sometimes the objection may be simply based on the perception that the body will have to remain for days at the morgue before its release. Usually, adequate communications with the family alleviates these fears and perceptions. The conversation should also deal with statutory requirements, the reason and necessity for the autopsy, and your concern for their feelings. It is essential to remember that while the autopsy may be routine for the pathologist, it is a very unique and emotional experience for the family.

If there is a personal objection in a case that clearly must be autopsied (e.g., homicide), a short preautopsy conference can greatly alleviate preconceived fears and apprehension. During this conference the requirements of the law are explained, along with the benefits to be gained by the family and society. In essence it is explained that the autopsy under these circumstances is done for the living and in the public interest. The family can also be reassured that only those procedures essential to the investigation will be performed and that, if possible, no organs will be removed. This short conference will generally go far in alleviating anxiety and assuaging the anger and fear of the grief reaction, which, temporarily, may be directed at the pathologist. A followup communication with the family is also helpful, in that they have the opportunity to ask questions and can be reassured (for example, that there was little or no suffering, no evidence of congenital disease, etc.). In a homicide case, however, one cannot relate specific details—such as the projectile pathway—without prior approval of the police or prosecuting attorney (particularly if a family member is a chief suspect!).

Some religions specifically prohibit the mutilation of a body, and others require that a person be buried intact. In either event, the religious belief may result in an objection to an autopsy. Unfortunately, there may be instances when the requirements of the law must supersede the religious wishes of the family. Usually, however, a compromise can be reached that will satisfy the requirements of the law and still respect the religious beliefs of the decedent and the family.

Religious objections are often from those of the Jewish faith. In essence, Jewish law prohibits ''Nivul ha-met,'' or the dishonoring of the dead. Furthermore, the body should be buried as quickly as possible. These two laws have been balanced by the duty of saving and maintaining life, ''Piku'ah Nefesh.'' Therefore, Judaism does permit autopsies in certain circumstances. While there is no universal agreement regarding when an autopsy may be performed, some rabbinical authorities have permitted postmortem examinations in the following circumstances:

1. if the autopsy is required by law (usually in homicide cases or when homicide is strongly suspected);
2. to determine the cause of death if it is uncertain and cannot be ascertained without autopsy;
3. to save a life;
4. to guide the family in instances of hereditary disease.

These have been formalized into a concordat entered between the chief rabbinate of Israel and Hadassah University Hospital.

When a religious concern or objection is expressed because of the Orthodox Jewish faith, we have found that a liaison with the local rabbinical council is beneficial to all concerned. After a discussion of the case with the pathologist, the rabbi explains the situation to the family, explains the religious tenets, assures them of the necessity for the autopsy, and assures them the autopsy will be performed in accordance with rabbinical law. The body is placed on a clean white sheet in an isolated area of the morgue. The only persons in attendance at the autopsy are those absolutely essential to the investigation: the pathologist, diener, police, and essential technicians. The autopsy is performed as expeditiously as possible (to permit rapid burial) and in the presence of the rabbi. An honor guard remains with the deceased until its release to the funeral home. The autopsy procedure is modified so that only the essential fluids are withdrawn for testing, minimal histologic sections are taken, and, if possible, no organs are removed. All procedures should be minimized insofar as possible, which often means an *in situ* dissection which is technically more difficult. A nearby plastic bag is used to receive all disposable items that come in contact with blood. Instruments are wiped off with paper towels and also placed in this bag, which is released to the funeral home for interment with the body along with the white sheet (the body is wrapped in this sheet after the autopsy).

The basic concept behind these guidelines revolves about the Jewish belief in the respect and dignity of the whole man. This tenet cannot be compromised, even after death. If a rabbi is not available, this procedure is almost invariably satisfactory to the Orthodox Jewish family, provided everything is explained to them beforehand. If the death occurs on the Jewish Sabbath, it is probably prudent to do nothing until the next day, since service work (including burial) cannot be done until then anyway.

The family should be given the option of receiving a phone call from the rabbi and/or medical examiner to discuss the results and their implications. Discourse between the medical examiner and the family after the autopsy can be highly productive not only in terms of the information provided, but also from the relief the truth may bring. For example, an instantaneous death due to a motor vehicle accident may well comfort family members who would not want their loved one to suffer from the pain of the incident. Such sessions with the family require sensitivity and skill on the part of the pathologist.

GENERAL PROCEDURES FOR POSTMORTEM EXAMINATION

Inprocessing

1. Upon arrival in the morgue, the body is immediately given an accession number. This, along with the name of the deceased, is recorded on a tag, which in turn is tied to the great toe.
2. The body is measured and weighed.
3. A photograph of the head and chest is taken with an accession number in the photograph. This photograph simply records the body as it was

received, and initiates identification of that body with that accession number.

4. Clothing and valuables are inventoried, recorded, and secured or given to the police or family as may be appropriate.
5. Fingerprints are taken.
6. Clothing is removed. However, in trauma cases, the clothing should not be removed until first inspected by the pathologist.
7. The body is cleaned.
8. The face is photographed again if the initial "as is" photograph recorded blood, dirt, etc.
9. The body is examined externally and all scars, marks, tattoos, injuries, etc. are recorded (sketched) on a body diagram. Always look at the back of the body!
10. All injuries are photographed.

These steps are carried out with every case that comes to our facility regardless of the apparent cause or manner of death, and whether or not an autopsy is to be performed. The identification procedures of fingerprints and photography are done even if identification of the victim is not in question. The minimal expenditure in cost and time may prove invaluable once the body is released. The most frequent problems the inprocessing procedures help alleviate are the following: when the next of kin wants visual proof that it was indeed their family member that died; in refuting allegations that facial distortions, injuries, or mutilation were caused by morgue personnel; and when there are allegations that the body was transported to the facility with jewelry or money which is now missing.

On rare occasions, information may surface after release of the body, or even after burial, that the death was really a homicide that was previously not suspected. The fingerprints and photographs in such circumstances are invaluable in averting the necessity of exhumation (which is time-consuming, expensive, and often emotionally impacts on the family). Should the body have been cremated, and no fingerprints or photographs were taken, positive identification may be impossible.

Whether or not an autopsy is anticipated, the body must be very carefully examined externally, since subtle findings may alter the course of the subsequent investigation. Specific attention should be paid to the following items, regardless of the apparent cause of death:

1. Carefully inspect the conjunctivae, mouth, and neck. The subtle external signs of strangulation may be manifested by conjunctival petechiae and minor abrasions or contusions of the neck. Bruises of the oral mucosa as well as a torn or contused frenulum may be the only anatomical

markers for smothering. Bitemarks of the lips, cheeks, or tongue may indicate terminal seizure activity that may or may not be consistent with the suspected cause of death.

2. Carefully inspect the scalp for any injury. Should a scalp injury be found, the area must be shaved, diagrammed, and photographed. Extensive injuries may require complete shaving of the scalp hair.
3. Look for wrist scars, or scars in the antecubital fossae, which might indicate prior suicide attempts.
4. Specifically check the mouth, lips, teeth, and hands for medication dye or pill residue that could indicate a drug overdose. Vomitus in the mouth or adherent to the face should also be examined for medication residue.
5. Look for needle puncture marks or scars that are not obviously iatrogenic.
6. Inspect the back no matter how innocuous or simple the case may seem. The small-caliber gunshot wound or ice pick stab wound may well be undetected if this practice is ignored. Bruises or abrasions of the back may have tremendous significance when the external examination is otherwise unremarkable. Some may indicate homicidal abuse of a child or elderly person. In one instance, a woman found next to a building was brought to an emergency room with an apparent heart attack. Blood pressure could never be sustained and she died. At the morgue, the back injuries were observed for the first time, and the autopsy led to further investigation that proved she had jumped from the building. *Always* look at the back carefully.

Create a System of Redundancy

The documentation of all medicolegal cases should have a purposely built-in system of redundancy. Should one aspect of documentation fail, backup sources of documentation will at least provide most of the information needed. Thus, body diagrams are invaluable as a backup source of documentation when the photographs do not come out, when the voice recorder fails, or when the autopsy report is misfiled! The photographs will settle questions such as orientation, for example, if the left to right direction of a projectile pathway is inadvertently reversed in the autopsy report or body diagrams. Thus, notes, diagrams, photographs, and the autopsy report all serve to complement each other and preserve information when something goes wrong. And sometimes one document may serve to correct an error in another document. Fingerprints, photographs, etc. do the same for identification purposes.

Consequently, liberal use should be made of photographs and body diagrams. These diagrams of various aspects of the human form have an advantage over photographs and the autopsy report in that they permit easier visualization of injury patterns and other characteristics. At a glance, all or at least most of the characteristic external features of a case are easily visualized. In some instances, these schematics may be made a part of the autopsy report for purposes of clarification, especially when there are multiple stab or gunshot wounds.

A Word About Photography

Adequate photographic documentation is essential for identification, legal purposes, consultation, and future review. All that is really required is any quality 35-mm camera with a flash attachment. It is recommended that an ultraviolet filter be placed over the lens to protect the lens and improve the color balance. For outdoor photography, a polarized filter will greatly improve the quality of the pictures. Color slide film is reasonably inexpensive and easy to process, and quality prints can readily be made from the slides if they are needed for legal purposes. The slides can be cheaply converted to Polaroid-type photographs with relatively inexpensive equipment available at most photography stores.

Each photograph should contain the accession number of the case. This should be placed to one side of the frame, not in the center. Rulers in the photograph generally serve more as a distraction than a provider of useful information, and hence are not very helpful (except for certain patterned injuries where closeup or one-to-one photographs are taken). Some recommend a color standard be included in the photographs. This again is usually more of a distraction than a provider of useful information, except in certain circumstances (e.g., bitemarks).

The area photographed should be clean and devoid of blood, instruments, and clutter. Although it is natural to concentrate on the area to be photographed when taking a picture, be sure also to check the periphery and background to eliminate clutter, distractions, etc. A photograph of an injury would not be admissible in court if blood and gore were depicted. The usual test is that the probative or demonstrative value of the photograph should outweigh any inflammatory or prejudicial aspects it might have.

When photographing injuries, two pictures are often needed—one taken at a distance to show where the injury is on the body, and a closer view to delineate the details of the injury. In general, photograph all identifying characteristics (face, scars, tattoos, etc.), all injuries, and blood or foreign material distribution if indicated (e.g., blood and gunpowder on a hand).

The Medicolegal Autopsy Procedure

The autopsy itself must be performed by the pathologist. Reliance on a diener for unobserved evisceration potentially introduces a second witness during subsequent legal proceedings and also may jeopardize the chain of custody. Legally, whatever the diener does or removes, and later relates to the pathologist, becomes hearsay evidence that may not be admissible in court. Objects with evidentiary value (e.g., projectiles) that are removed by the diener interposes another link in the custody chain. The pathologist has sole responsibility for the case and will be the primary witness as to the cause of death as well as the evidentiary aspects of the case. Consequently, it is imperative that the pathologist be the one to perform the external examination, *in situ* inspection, evisceration, and removal and preservation of objects with evidentiary value. The diener is relegated to the role of an assistant under the direct supervision of the pathologist. In our practice the diener may only reflect the scalp and, after direct inspection by the pathologist, open (best not remove) the calvarium.

Following the usual Y-shaped incision, the body cavities and organs are inspected *in situ*. At this point, obtain all fluids necessary for toxicologic testing (usually blood from the heart or aorta, bile, urine, and ocular fluid). Routinely doing this at the beginning ensures that the specimens are in hand and not forgotten or inadvertently lost. As they are placed in their previously labeled containers, the assistant must show the label to the prosector, who must stop what other activty is being done and actively look at the label. Assuming the label is correct, reading the label before the autopsy, or having the label read to you is courting the dangers of a serious error.

Organs are then removed via a modified Virchow technique—i.e., organ by organ, or by related blocks of organs. We prefer this over the Rokitansky technique, since injury patterns and projectile pathways are more easily followed and delineated. Also, the pathologist must be actively thinking of directions and relationships, such as right to left, back to front, etc. This has proven to be much easier with the modified Virchow procedure, since, with the Rokitansky technique, the dissection is via a posterior approach.

What constitutes a "complete" autopsy is usually a matter of individual philosophy and the subject of fruitless discussion. However, one should keep in mind that the medicolegal autopsy, particularly where the manner of death is not natural, is problem-oriented and directed toward the answering of future questions, most of which should be anticipated. At the very minimum, all major organs (including the brain and neck organs) should be removed and dissected. The dura mater is routinely removed to permit inspection of the skull for fractures or other abnormalities (one should never rely solely on X-rays, even if they are taken and interpreted by a radiologist). As a practical course, the pancreas, internal genitalia, adrenal glands, and thyroid gland may usually be inspected and dissected *in situ* unless otherwise indicated. All necessary dissections must be performed that address the issues of a particular case. This includes areas not routinely dissected, such as the tendons of the wrist, the back of the neck, or wherever necessary information is to be obtained.

Stomach contents should always be carefully inspected, since this may be the first clue that the death was from drug ingestion and was not, as originally suspected, from natural disease. The amount and type of food in the stomach not infrequently becomes important to police or family members when they inquire about time of death, what was last eaten, etc.

With most trauma cases it is usually not necessary to take a large number of histologic sections, as would be typical for the usual hospital autopsy. However, it is imperative that sections meaningfully document the necessary aspects of the case. A section of a normal (or diseased) coronary artery would be indicated in the death of a motor vehicle crash victim (particularly if the victim was the driver). Likewise a section of the margin of a suicidal gunshot wound would document the presence of gunpowder, and a section of the liver may help answer future questions concerning chronic alcoholism.

Toxicology

The specimens to be taken for toxicologic analysis are largely determined by the nature of the case. In all deaths, a 10-ml sample of blood (obtained from the heart or aorta), and preserved with sodium fluoride, is obtained. The sodium fluoride inhibits bacterial growth and thereby prevents a spurious elevation of alcohol. Also, it inhibits certain enzymes (e.g., cholinesterase), which could artificially lower the levels of some drugs such as cocaine. This "retainer tube" sample is refrigerated and kept indefinitely (space and facilities permitting), should subsequent information indicate the necessity of toxicologic testing.

Deaths from trauma of any kind should have blood, urine, and ocular fluid taken (if no urine is available, washing of the urinary bladder may be helpful). The urine is subjected to a screening test for drugs. If a drug is detected in the urine, it should be quantified in the blood, since questions often arise as to how a drug may have influenced the victim's behavior. Alcohol should be measured in both the blood and the ocular fluid. The latter serves to confirm the validity of the blood alcohol concentration and may be helpful if intravenous fluids were given, if the victim was in an early absorptive phase, or when there may be an artificial increase in blood alcohol because of decomposition or a ruptured stomach. Depending on the circumstances of the case, it may also be advisable to obtain a second blood sample from a peripheral source, such as the femoral vein. In traumatic deaths, it is recommended that the following specimens be obtained:

Blood—10 ml in fluoride preservative ("retainer tube")

Blood—50 ml in fluoride preservative (for immediate testing)

Blood—10 ml with no preservative (if blood grouping or enzyme typing is necessary)

Ocular fluid—All from both eyes, in fluoride preservative (for alcohol content); use an 18- or 20-gauge needle, since the vitreous humor may be quite viscous; do not use a preservative if the ocular fluid is to be analyzed for electrolytes.

Urine—All available up to 50 ml (no preservative) for drug screening.

In trauma victims where the heart or aorta is lacerated, one has no recourse but to obtain blood from the chest cavity. The validity of the alcohol concentration in this sample could be challenged, hence the importance of obtaining the ocular fluid and a sample of peripheral blood outside the abdominal cavity. Also, 8–10 ml of blood usually remains in the pulmonary trunk even when the aorta has been transected; this sample would provide a better result for alcohol concentration than the chest blood.

Blood from the heart or great vessels should be obtained with a syringe with a 14-gauge needle. Always fill the container without a preservative ("red top") first, since accidental contamination of this sample with sodium fluoride will interfere with enzyme typing. If blood cannot be obtained by syringe because of postmortem clots, use the pericardial trapping technique: open the pericardial sac, dry it with a towel, sever the great vessels, and collect the blood that accumulates.

If there is a suspicion of recent drug ingestion, the entire stomach contents should be saved along with the contents of the small bowel to determine the amount of unabsorbed drug. Liver (100–300 gm) and bile (in fluoride preservative) may also be retained if there is a suspicion of chronic drug ingestion or of narcotic abuse. When placing the specimens into their containers, be sure that they are already labeled. Once the specimen is put in the container and the container is closed, we require that the label be shown to the prosector. Having an assistant read the label or simply checking it at the end of the autopsy may readily lead to embarrassing and serious errors.

Circumstances may dictate that other specimens be obtained. Whenever a death occurs in a hospital but the medical examiner or coroner has jurisdiction, admission samples of blood, urine, and gastric lavage should be obtained. Swabs of the nose should be obtained in cases of suspected cocaine users (sometimes opiate users may also "snort" heroin or other narcotics). In cases of suspected intravenous drug abuse, the injection sites (skin and subcutaneous fat) should be submitted for toxicologic analysis. Some poisons (e.g., herbicides, pesticides, inhalants, heavy metals, organic solvents, automotive coolants, etc.) may require other specimens such as brain, lung, fat, or kidney. If possible, check with a toxicologist before proceeding with the autopsy on a suspected case of environmental poisoning.

Cyanide is volatile and may decrease in a sample of blood. Hence, when testing for cyanide is important, the sample should be given to the laboratory without delay and it should be tested as soon as possible. Also, not everyone can smell cyanide. Those who can, describe a peculiar and distinctive odor that is detectable even at the autopsy in cases of poisoning. It is prudent to find out who among your staff can smell this chemical. A bottle of sodium ferricyanide smells like ammonia to those who cannot detect cyanide.

THE HOMICIDE VICTIM

In addition to the usual inprocessing procedures, the homicide victim requires special attention in two areas: (1) identification and (2) preservation of evidence with a documented chain of custody.

Identification

The identification of the homicide victim is more formal and stringent than in most other cases. In part this is because it forms part of the *corpus delicti* that is presented by the state during the criminal trial. The first part of the *corpus delicti* is that the person killed was indeed that individual, and the second is that the death resulted from a criminal action. Both must be proved to the exclusion of every reasonable doubt. Hence the basis for the "legal identification." This not only applies to the obvious homicide victim but also to those victims of automobile crashes or other injuries where the manner of death is certified as accidental but where manslaughter charges may be filed. Also, it should be remembered that death from recreational drug use (heroin, cocaine, phencyclidine, etc.) may result in third-degree murder charges in some jurisdictions. When in doubt get the legal identification.

In most cases the legal identification is accomplished by allowing an acquaintance of the deceased to view the body and sign a brief statement that it is indeed the remains of the individual known during life. It is perhaps best to do this with someone who is not a direct family member (to reduce the likelihood of emotional outbursts). Since most morgue facilities (especially in hospitals) are not designed for such viewing, a Polaroid photograph of the victim may be used.

In actual practice, we request the family or police to have an acquaintance come to the office to identify the deceased. Polaroid photographs of the deceased (frontal and lateral views with the accession number included in the picture) are taken after the body has been cleaned but before the autopsy is begun. The acquaintance then views the pictures and confirms the identity of the victim. The photographs are signed by the acquaintance and a typed statement is prepared. This statement provides the full name, address, telephone number, and driver's license number (or other form of identification) of the acquaintance, a sentence stating that the deceased was known to the acquaintance as "N," and the signature of the acquaintance. Naturally, the date, time, and accession number are included on the statement as well as the signature of a witness who was present during the identification (secretary, police officer, doctor, investigator, etc.).

If the identification is made by directly viewing the body, this should be photographically documented. This photograph should include the acquaintance, the face of the victim, and the accession number.

Fingerprints of the victim may also serve as a legal identification, provided fingerprints are already on record with some governmental agency. Severely mutilated bodies, decomposed bodies, and skeletal remains require special procedures for identification. These include fingerprints (if obtainable), dental identification (i.e., comparison of dentition with existing dental records), or radiologic examination. Most of these procedures are beyond the expertise of most pathologists and require the attention and testimony of other specialists.

Legal identification of children is done in much the same fashion, except that footprints must be taken. This is necessary even in cases of infanticide to preclude the possibility of double jeopardy. In some locales, schools or other organizations may take fingerprints of children as part of a program to identify missing children. Hence, if a child is unknown, it is best to take both footprints and fingerprints.

Evidence and Chain of Custody

Physical evidence may be anything taken from the scene or victim. Clothing, knives, guns, bullets, toxicology specimens, and even photographs may constitute physical evidence. Not only must the evidence be preserved, it must be accounted for in terms of who or what agency had possession of the item and for what purpose. The people who handled the evidence along the way are links in the so-called chain of custody. In legal parlance, the chain of custody is called *authenticating* the evidence, laying a proper *predicate* or *foundation* for exhibiting the items during the trial.

Most items obtained during the autopsy will be turned over to others for transportation, analysis, or storage until the trial. Hence, to ensure there is no mixup or alteration of the items, the samples are treated like a registered letter: each person who handles the item signs a piece of paper attached to the item with an indication as to the reason (date and time are also included). The person from whom the specimen is received is given a receipt as the custody changes hands. The vehicle or instrument used to record the chain of custody is known as a property receipt. Police agencies already have these forms and they may be used. If they are not available, one can easily make up a form.

All property receipts should document the following:

1. Name of the decedent.
2. Date and time of collection.
3. Accession number.
4. Name and signature of person who collected the item.

5. Item(s)—(Numbered 1, 2, 3, etc.)
   Note: Many items may be listed on one property receipt. However, bear in mind that if listed together, the items must stay together. Thus, it is best to fill out separate receipts for items that will go to different laboratories or agencies.
6. Signature of person receiving the item.
7. Reason for transfer.
8. Date and time of transfer.
   Note: Since several transfers may be anticipated, several lines should be included for the items 6 through 8.

Any item which is to pass from one agency to another must be accompanied by a property receipt. However, it is not necessary that a property receipt be filled out for each transfer of material within a department. This is because of the legal presumption that no hospital or government employee has altered the evidence, and this includes laboratory specimens or other sealed evidence containers. The presumption is predicated on the documentation as to who collected and sealed the specimen, who broke the seal for testing purposes, and that the specimen was in substantially the same condition as when collected.

The evidence most commonly sent to an outside agency for testing or storage is serology and toxicology specimens, bullets, trace evidence, and clothing. These specimens must be properly packaged and labeled. Each sample must have a label that not only links it to that particular case but also identifies who put the specimen in the container and who took it out for testing. The specimen container, whether it be a test tube, envelope, or paper bag, should be labeled with the decedent's name (if known), autopsy number, date and time of collection, and contents. The pathologist should sign the label and attach the specimen to the property receipt. When the specimen is removed for testing or examination, the technologist should initial the label and note the date and time.

The method of evidence collection will vary depending on circumstances. For example, a shirt with bullet holes is sometimes collected directly at the scene, whereas the bullet is obtained at the autopsy or afterward.

Clothing

Clothing with evidentiary value should first be photographed and then removed from the victim. If bloody or wet, it should be dried before it is transferred to the police. If the clothing contains important serologic evidence (blood, seminal stains), care must be exercised to avoid contamination. These specimens should be collected from the clothing first, and then the items should be cut off the body with a pinking shears. After air drying, each item should be individually wrapped in plain paper. Never use plastic wrapping or plastic containers, since these retain moisture and promote microbial and fungal growth.

Trace Evidence

Trace evidence such as glass, plastic, paint chips, and hairs may be placed in small labeled envelopes and stapled to the property receipt. The specimens should be dry to avoid microbial growth. The test tube is ideal for very small specimens, which can often be removed from the victim or clothing with the tip of the ever-present scalpel. The scalpel itself may be deposited in the test tube if the sample sticks to the blade. Alternatively, tiny specimens of glass or paint may stick to clear adhesive tape and be submitted in an envelope.

Bullets

When the autopsy is completed and the projectiles are sorted out, they must be appropriately marked (except shotshell pellets) at the base or nose with the case number and initials of the pathologist (if there is enough room). If space is limited, the last two digits of the case number or the pathologist's initials may be inscribed. A vibrating engraving device works well for inscribing. If the projectile (or projectile fragment) is deformed or small, simply do not mark it. Dry off the projectile, photograph it with the accession number, and place it in a small labeled envelope, which is then sealed and stapled to a property receipt. Projectile fragments from the same gunshot wound may be placed in a single envelope. However, if there is a chance that metal contacting metal may alter the rifling features, the fragments should be submitted separately (e.g., the case of the bullet and the jacket in separate envelopes). The envelope label should state what is inside and where it was found [e.g., ''projectile from (R) chest cavity'', ''projectile fragments (5) from cranial vault'']. It is prudent to write on the envelope how the projectile was inscribed (e.g., ''projectile inscribed 917 RM at base''). This may save time in court when you are asked if this is the bullet removed from a particular victim, since these inscriptions are often difficult to read. The uniqueness of the evidence is further verified by the description on the property receipt. If the item is listed as ''brown envelope with projectile removed from the head,'' then the envelope and the projectile must stay together. The envelope, then, with proper labeling and your signature is further proof that this was indeed the projectile removed from the victim. Another excellent way to assist in projectile identification, even years later, is to simply photograph the bullet with the labeled envelope into which the bullet is to be placed.

Summary

Common sense must prevail in preserving evidence and documenting the chain of custody. The goal is to enable you, at trial, to:

1. Identify the specimen as the one you collected on a specific date;
2. State definitely from whom the item was taken;

3. State that it is in substantially the same condition now as when you collected it.

Only when the above criteria are met can the courts be sure that the evidence is properly preserved and documented. This allows for it to be admitted into evidence and therefore provides the data base upon which expert witness testimony can be rendered.

AFTER THE AUTOPSY

The Autopsy Protocol and the English Language

Since medicolegal autopsies are performed in the public interest, the work product (namely, the autopsy report) is frequently not guarded by the rules of patient confidentiality common to hospital records. These reports will be read by attorneys, insurance adjustors, and then nonmedical personnel including family members. Consequently, the report should be intelligible to the lay person as much as possible. This means it should be easily read, address the issues of the particular case with pertinent observations and appropriate ''pertinent negatives,'' and be free of excess medical jargon.

The autopsy report should also reflect the professionalism of the physician who made that report. It should be in good polished English, grammatically correct, and devoid of medical slang. Avoidance of the following expressions will vastly improve the readability of the autopsy report and project the professionalism of the pathologist:

Avoid beginning sentences with *There is* or *There are*. Some authors begin well over 75% of their sentences with either of these expressions, and the habit is hard to break because it is convenient albeit meaningless. Instead of saying ''There is a gunshot would of the chest . . .'' simply start with the subject of the sentence: ''A gunshot wound of the chest . . .''

Avoid medical *slang*. The ''LAD'' is really the anterior descending branch of the left coronary artery. This is much more intelligible to a lay person than LAD. The ''right heart,'' ''left chest,'' etc. imply two separate and distinct hearts or chests. The left or right side (or aspect) is more precise. An ''IV line'' is really a vascular or intravenous catheter.

Avoid *redundant expressions:* ''The liver is *brown* in *color,*'' ''The right lung *weighs* 400 *gm,*'' ''cut section,'' ''rubbery in *consistency*'' are but a few examples. Simply state the modifier: ''the 400-gm right lung,'' ''the brown liver,'' ''the gray, rubbery tumor,'' etc. Instead of ''cut section,'' say the ''cut surface'' or ''upon sectioning.'' The terms ''is present,'' ''is noted,'' and ''is evident'' do nothing but take up space. Thus ''A gunshot wound is present on the chest'' should simply be ''a gunshot wound of the chest.'' The phrase ''without note'' is a poor way of saying ''essentially normal,'' which should also be avoided (see below).

PROPERTY RECEIPT

DADE COUNTY MEDICAL EXAMINER DEPARTMENT
1050 N.W. 19th Street
Miami, Florida 33136

(305) 549-7337

M.E. CASE # ____________

MEDICAL EXAMINER ____________

(IF NOT KNOWN, USE UNK)

DECEDENT'S NAME: ____________

AGE ______ RACE ______ SEX ______ TYPE OF CASE ____________

POLICE AGENCY: ____________ POLICE CASE # ______

ITEM NO.	QUANTITY	**DESCRIPTION** (itemize currency by denomination)

I hereby acknowledge that the above list represents all the property impounded by me in the official performance of my duty as Medical Examiner, District 11.

____________ Print ____________ Sign

DATE/TIME OBTAINED: ____________ MO. DAY YR. ____________AM./PM TIME

I hereby acknowledge that the above list represents all property received by/from the Medical Examiner Department.

M.E. Courier: ____________ Print ____________ Sign

DATE/TIME OBTAINED: ____________ MO DAY YR. ____________ AM./PM. TIME

Receiving Party: ____________ Print ____________ Sign ______ Agency

Date & Time Released: ____________ MO. DAY YR. ____________ AM./PM. TIME

Reason: ____________

____

____

____

Avoid *irrelevant observations*. In a normal 21-year-old male who died of a gunshot wound of the heart, it is irrelevant to say that the testes are descended bilaterally, the renal capsules strip with ease, and the scalp hair is 3½ inches long. When the time of death is not in question, the mentioning of fixed lividity or the degree of rigor mortis is also not needed and just adds useless verbiage to the protocol. Should any of these or similar phrases, observations, or descriptions actually be pertinent to a particular case, they should obviously be mentioned.

Avoid *references to procedures*. Nobody cares that "The body is opened with the standard Y-shaped incision," or that "The heart is dissected in the direction of blood flow." Autopsy procedures should only be mentioned if they convey something specific to the reader. To specifically indicate that the dura mater is stripped from the skull and calvarium indicates the bones of the skull were directly visualized by the prosector (and by inference, therefore, that a fracture was in fact not present). A procedural statement that the popliteal fossae and femoral triangles were dissected tells the reader that the prosector actually searched for the source of a fatal pulmonary thromboembolism.

Avoid *shows, reveals,* or *demonstrates*. These terms reflect an activity of the prosector, not of an organ. The cut surface of the liver does not show (or reveal or demonstrate) a pattern of chronic passive congestion. It is more correct to say "The liver *is* brown" or "The liver *has* a pattern of chronic passive congestion." "Sectioning reveals . . ." would be correct, since the phrase reflects a procedure or action of the prosector.

Avoid *hemorrhage*. Although firmly entrenched in medical jargon, hemorrhage actually refers to the active flow of blood. At autopsy one sees extravasated blood, the *result* of hemorrhage. It is therefore more precise and objective simply to say that blood is in the subarachnoid space, or that the leptomeninges and subarachnoid space are hemorrhagic.

Avoid *essentially normal*. In the case of a normal 21-year-old male who died of a gunshot wound of the head, it is tempting simply to list the organ weights and say that all the enumerated organs were "essentially normal." This statement saves time, typing, and effort and it is also true: the organs are essentially normal, at least insofar as they are free of any intrinsic diseases. However, there are three very real problems with this expression. First, it leaves the reader in doubt as to whether these organs were, in fact examined thoroughly. Second, it fails to address the morphologic expression of the pathophysiologic process (mechanism) leading to death. Normal organs respond in a variety of ways to trauma and pathophysiologic events, and these are often manifested in a variety of morphologic alterations. These must be described both as to their appearance and as to what they do or do not have. In the case of the gunshot wound of the head, it is pertinent to note the presence or absence of aspirated blood, pulmonary edema, pallor of the liver, etc. Third, it encourages the pathologist to gloss over observations that may have importance to others yet have nothing to do with the cause of death. Family members and others frequently inquire as to the presence or absence of diseases, signs of the early development of certain diseases (e.g., atherosclerosis), the residual of prior diseases (e.g., rheumatic fever), the explanation for certain complaints during life (e.g., intermittent chest pain), and the potential for a long life. The "essentially normal" heart, with mild or moderate coronary arteriosclerosis, takes on added significance when it is subsequently learned that all males in a family died of heart attacks before the age of 45 years. Since one frequently does not know the significance of minor structural alterations at the time of the autopsy, it is best to describe them to tell the reader you actually did your job and individualized the case. Morphologic alterations resulting from the mechanism of death are recorded, and the pathologist can more readily and intelligently answer unanticipated questions as they arise.

The dictated autopsy report, therefore, should specifically address the major issues of the case, anticipate questions that may not have anything to do with the cause of death, and be obviously individualized. The report should be readable and easily understood. Subsequently, less time will be devoted to translating medical jargon and explaining what should be obvious.

At times it becomes necessary to retain certain organs for a more detailed dissection after a period of formalin fixation. Even though this would be legally permissible under most jurisdictions, any reference to organ retention should be avoided in the autopsy report. The main reason for this is to avoid consternation on the part of family members. As a practical matter, most people would prefer to have accurate answers than to read about what was actually done to their loved one. Naturally, should the question be directly posed as to whether the heart or brain was saved for further study, one would have to honestly acknowledge that fact. Rarely, the family may wish to have these returned for interment for religious or personal reasons.

The Autopsy Protocol: Format

The usual format for the hospital autopsy report is designed to elucidate disease processes and provide a clinicopathological correlation. The medicolegal autopsy report must, of necessity, have a different format, since it often addresses injuries that must be correlated with a terminal event.

In the usual hospital setting, the autopsy concludes the inquiry of the patient's medical course and death. The medicolegal autopsy is performed in the midst of an ongoing investigation, and on occasion may even initiate an investigation. The initial information provided on a medicolegal case may be incomplete or even erroneous. Also, the investigation by the police, crime laboratory, and others (including the pathologist) usually continues for some time after the autopsy is completed. Consequently, interpretation and conclusions may change as more information becomes available. For these reasons, then, the medicolegal autopsy report should be a completely objective document that allows for varying interpretations as more information becomes available. The only interpretive or high-level conclusion that should appear in the report is the cause of death (as it appears on the death certificate).

It is recommended that each page of the report include the name of the decedent (if known) along with any known aliases, the date and time of the autopsy, and the accession number. In the format we use, the first page has only the cause of death, the typed name and signature of the pathologist, and the date the report was completed. The next page is the toxicology report, which is initialed or signed by the pathologist with the date that it was reviewed by the pathologist. The next page begins the autopsy report itself. This is preceded by a brief sentence or two providing information about the legal identification of the victim, if this was actually done. At the end of the report is a list of autopsy findings (see below) and the signature of the pathologist. Sometimes a body diagram that schematically locates numerous injuries (such as multiple gunshot wounds) will greatly clarify the autopsy report. This is actually attached to the end of the report, and therefore also becomes a part of the official autopsy report.

Conspicuously absent from the report is a synopsis of the history or terminal event, and an "epicrisis" or clinicopathological correlation. A description of the clothing may be included in the report. In some medical examiner offices, a detailed clothing description is included with every autopsy report. In others, including this one, a detailed clothing description is done only if it has a particular importance to the case (e.g., an unidentified victim, or if the clothing helps the interpretation of entrance or exit gunshot wounds, etc.). In such cases, the clothing description generally appears elsewhere in the case file, but not in the autopsy report.

For ease of reading, and for easy reference when you are on the witness stand, several major headings and the liberal use of paragraphs (double-spaced from the preceding paragraph) are essential. Since most Americans do not understand the metric system, it is generally preferable to indicate external measurements in inches instead of centimeters. As a practical matter, you will probably be ordered to convert the metric system into inches anyway at a deposition or on the witness stand, so using inches to begin with prevents annoying calculations at a later time. All descriptions refer to the standard anatomic position. For the body of the autopsy report, the following format is recommended.

Legal Identification

If this was done, include the name of the person who identified the deceased, his or her driver's license number or other identifier, relation to the deceased (e.g., friend for 5 years), address, telephone number, the date and time of the identification, and the name of whoever witnessed the identification.

External Examination

This is the overall external appearance of the decedent but *without* the inclusion of any injuries or terminal medical intervention. The idea here is to provide a verbal picture of the victim as he or she would have appeared before any injury or resuscitative attempts occurred. Race, sex, height, weight, apparent age, hair color, etc. are included. Scars and tattoos must be mentioned but detailed descriptions are generally not needed unless there is a potential problem with identification or unique aspects of a case would warrant such detail (e.g. tattoos indicative of gang associations).

Evidence of Medical Intervention

In this paragraph, the placement of all vascular catheters, tubes, etc. is described. To avoid redundancy later in the report, include a phrase to indicate whether or not these items were properly placed. For example: "An endotracheal tube, a urinary catheter, and an intravenous catheter in the left antecubital fossa are all subsequently seen to be properly positioned. A nasogastric tube is subsequently found to be coiled upon itself in the upper esophagus behind the cuff of the endotracheal tube." Likewise, rib and sternal fractures resulting from resuscitative efforts are included here, along with exploratory surgical alterations.

Evidence of Injury

All major and minor injuries are described. Make liberal use of paragraphs and organize the paragraphs so that the minor injuries of one area are described, then another area, etc. Then describe the major injuries as to what the injury is (e.g., entrance-type gunshot wound), general location (e.g., right side of the head), specific location (e.g., 2 inches above and behind external ear canal), and the external dimensions and appearance of the wound itself. The wound is then traced through to its completion (e.g., gunshot wound through the skull, brain, and other side of the skull, and exit-type wound with the location and external appearance as for the entrance gunshot wound). Any other findings associated with this injury are also described (e.g., "The wound is associated with multiple fractures of the floor of the anterior cranial fossa and blood in the sphenoid sinus"). The final sentence should be a brief general summary of the direction of the wound path (e.g., "The projectile pathway is right to left, front to back, and slightly upward").

Internal Examination

In this section, the body cavities and organs are described as to their appearance, but excluding injuries or alterations created by resuscitative attempts. On occasion, it may be necessary to include a reference to an injury just so the report sounds sensible (e.g., "Aside from the previously described laceration, the 1500-gm liver . . .").

At the conclusion of the internal examination, one may wish to note the presence of any unusual odors from alcohol, drugs, or poisons. Since the toxicology laboratory is far better than the nose at identifying and quantifying such substances, it is best to keep the description objective, or if highly characteristic, an indication as to what it might be (e.g., ''During the autopsy a sweet aromatic odor reminiscent of alcohol is detected'').

Autopsy Findings

This is simply a list of the major injuries, diseases, and abnormalities observed at the autopsy table. In a barbiturate overdose, the autopsy findings may be nothing more than pulmonary edema and generalized visceral congestion. An otherwise normal individual who died from a gunshot wound of the chest would simply have ''penetrating (or perforating) gunshot wound of the chest'' as the autopsy finding. Findings associated with injuries (e.g., hemothorax) need not be listed. Conclusions based upon historical knowledge of the case should not be listed. Thus, one might describe an enlarged, yellow, greasy liver with a rounded anterior edge. The autopsy finding would be listed as severe fatty metamorphosis (or fatty change) of the liver. The conclusion is an expressed opinion as to what was responsible for the liver alteration—idiopathic hepatic steatosis, chronic alcoholism, etc. This conclusion may be expressed on the death certificate or rendered as an interpretive opinion at a legal proceeding. But alcoholism is not an autopsy finding.

The format described for the body of the autopsy report works quite well for all cases except those with multiple injuries from falls or from vehicular crashes. In those instances the format is modified slightly. The Evidence of Injury heading is changed to External Evidence of Injury, and the internal injuries are incorporated into the Internal Examination section. Instead of listing all the injuries in such cases, the autopsy findings are usually general (e.g., ''multiple injuries of head, chest, and lower extremities'').

Residency training in autopsy pathology requires the pathologist to think in terms of organ systems and anatomic regions, and the autopsy report is organized accordingly. Consequently, there is the temptation to describe all injuries by anatomic region. In trauma victims this often leads to immense confusion and an unintelligible autopsy report. Therefore, when a victim has numerous and varied injuries, organize the Evidence of Injury section into an appropriate number of subheadings of injury types. In the case of a woman who was raped and murdered, the following subheadings may appear: Stab Wounds, Incised Wounds, Blunt Force Injuries, and Evidence of Strangulation.

Finally, an additional heading entitled Evidence Collection may be interposed between the Evidence of Injury and Internal Examination sections. This would simply list what materials were collected for evidentiary purposes or subsequent testing that would not otherwise be stated in the autopsy report. Projectiles from gunshot wounds would normally be mentioned with the description of the gunshot wound, but scalp and pubic hair standards, swabs for spermatozoa and acid phosphatase, etc. would not. Such out-of-the-ordinary procedures could therefore be mentioned in this section. We usually do not include an Evidence Collection section, since copies of the property receipts or the laboratory reports (or both) are included in the case file. Depending on circumstances or philosophy, you may nevertheless find this section (with its built-in redundancy) quite useful.

Funeral Homes

Unfortunately, medicolegal autopsies sometimes require fairly mutilating dissections. This is particularly true in cases of child abuse, where the eyes may be removed and multiple incisions made on the back, and in cases of multiple gunshot wounds where projectiles are difficult to locate. Although only the hands and the head and neck of the deceased are generally exposed while in repose, the funeral director must be concerned about leakage of embalming fluid. Consequently, necessary but mutilating dissection complicates the work of the funeral director. However, their job can be made a bit easier if they are simply informed of the problem before they begin their embalming procedure. Obviously, tying off large vessels that were severed is helpful, as is leaving the aorta and aortic arch intact insofar as possible. If ocular fluid is withdrawn for toxicologic or electrolyte determination, the eyes should be injected with formalin. Telling the funeral director what extra incisions were made and why provides for cooperation and an understanding of each other's problems. Communication is essential.

Often overlooked is the fact that funeral home personnel are exposed to a variety of diseases. Consequently it is important to alert them to the presence of any evident or suspected diseases that may be a biohazard. Many times these do not appear on a death certificate. A person who died of a self-inflicted gunshot wound because he was depressed after receiving a diagnosis of AIDS would be a biohazard for funeral home personnel. Although revealing the diagnosis of AIDS may be a breach of medical confidentiality, the funeral director should be informed that "hepatitis precautions" are needed in handling the body. The same would hold true for the unexpected discovery of caseous granulomas or the fact that a person was an intravenous drug abuser, regardless of the actual cause of death.

The Case File

The case file is simply a large (12 × 14 inches) envelope that contains virtually all the paperwork and photographs (35-mm slides in plastic pages and legal identification photographs). Included are fingerprint cards, property receipts, the autopsy report, newspaper articles, subpoenas, medical records, police reports, body diagrams, and notes of conversations and telephone calls made or received.

In medicolegal cases it is imperative that all activity concerning a particular case be documented with the time and date. Activity includes telephone and personal conversations, the examination of equipment, consultation, etc. Such notes can be variously detailed, depending on the circumstances. The main point is that a continuous record must be kept. The reason is that future inquiries, be they informal or at a deposition, may well center about how conclusions were made and the source of the information. In short, these notes with documented dates and times are invaluable when the case comes to trial a year or more after the autopsy is done.

Copies of body diagrams or other documents are frequently given to police or attorneys, or introduced as evidence during a trial. Initial the original document with red or blue ink to be sure you get the original back.

What is confidential in the case file, what is public record, and what is regarded as a work product (and therefore public record) will be largely determined by law. In this jurisdiction, the entire case file, including notes and the autopsy report, is considered as public record, except for items that were confidential prior to being included in the file. Thus, medical records preserve their confidentiality, even though a copy of these records is included in the file. As with medical records in general, an attorney or other citizen would have to obtain a court order to get a copy. Included as medical records are records of telephone conversations between a treating physician, such as a psychiatrist, and the pathologist. In practice, these notes are covered with a separate sheet of paper indicating their confidentiality.

Not infrequently, opposing attorneys may request a conference regarding an individual case. Since the records you keep of these discussions may reveal the theory or trial tactic of one attorney, these notes should be kept confidential and not revealed to the other attorney. In practice, one set of notes is labeled plaintiff (or prosecuting) attorney notes, and the other, defense attorney notes. Both attorneys are aware of the existence of these notes, and it would be regarded as unethical to reveal a theory or the notes to an opposing attorney. This preserves the neutrality of your eventual testimony and allows you to be a better witness, since you are familiar with what the attorneys are trying to elicit (e.g., various possible scenarios to account for a pattern of gunshot wounds). These notes also protect you, since they are a record of theories and questions and your response to those questions. Hence, should there be an accusation that you purposely misled one attorney, these records will become invaluable in explaining your response to questions on the witness stand. Rarely, one attorney may insist that your notes with an opposing attorney are a work product (and therefore public record) and he or she has a right to examine these notes. Should the opposing attorney object to this, it then becomes a legal matter: is it a work product and is it unethical to reveal these notes? In this situation it is best to allow the attorneys to argue their points before a judge, and then simply abide by the court's decision.

The entire case file is kept confidential any time there is a homicide, or suspected homicide, under active investigation. It becomes public record once an indictment is made. Should the investigation become no longer active, then the file would become public record. Again, laws vary as to what is or is not subject to public scrutiny. When in doubt, it is best to get a written authorization from the police and/or state attorney (district attorney or U.S. magistrate) before releasing the file to another interested party.

News Media

Members of the news media may be interested in nearly any violent death in a community. A murder in a small town would perhaps be front-page news, whereas the same incident in a large city may go virtually unnoticed. In any location, news media will generally be interested in disasters, the death of a prominent person, any death that is particularly tragic (e.g., a child starved to death), and any death that has some sensational aspect (multiple killings, torture murder, murder in a hospital, etc.). Reporters may appear at any time singly, sequentially, or *en masse*. Their basic philosophy is that the public has a right to know about events occuring in their community, and that the information should be timely, factual, and accurate. The job of the reporter is to "get it fast, get it right, and get it first." This frequently imparts a sense of urgency (real or imagined) and therefore pressures police, coroners, and medical examiners for the immediate release of information. Some coroners or medical examiners simply refuse to talk to the news media and refer everything to a police spokesperson (larger jurisdictions often have a designated public information officer). Others are readily willing to provide information to the press, provided the information is appropriate, not premature, and not speculative, and that the release of this information does not interfere with an ongoing criminal investigation.

Assuming you are willing to talk with the news media, there are certain ground rules that must be observed. In our view, talking with the news media is merely a "part of the job." Under no circumstances should the news media be a vehicle for ego gratification or personal aggrandizement. Comments must be restricted to your area of expertise and to the pertinent facts of the case based upon your observation and test results. This means that questions regarding background information and terminal events are to be referred to other sources even if you know the answers. It would be inappropriate, for example, to comment on the details of a love triangle that led to a murder. Such information should be released by the police or another appropriate agency. If a question appears inappropriate (e.g., "What are your personal feelings . . ."), simply decline to comment or diplomatically skirt the question. Finally, no media interview should be given without first consulting with the investigating police agency as to what information may or may not be released. In obvious or suspected cases of homicide, they may request that you say nothing and refer all inquiries to them, or they may permit the release of limited information. Sometimes they may simply request a delay in the release of information until they can positively identify the victim.

Situations attracting national attention (e.g., mass disaster or a bizarre murder) may present with the sudden appearance of a multitude of reporters with note pads and microphones in hand and accompanied by a host of technicians and video cameras. This usually occurs at the scene of death, and if you are in the spotlight the main problem is one of control. The first priority is to stop the hail of questions, and then release to all whatever information is appropriate. Following that, answer only one question at a time, only after being sure you understand the question. Conclude by indicating that more information will be released as it becomes available, and, if possible, give an approximate time when they should call your office.

Even if there is no streetside interview with numerous reporters, these situations bring a barrage of telephone calls. Again, control is of paramount importance to allow you and your staff to function and, at the same time, provide appropriate information as it becomes available. This control can usually be obtained by designating only one person to release information. First, all office personnel are to be instructed that no information is to be released to anybody except by the designated representative. This could be yourself, an administrator, or an investigator. Initially it is probably best to designate the administrator or investigator. Second, have typed a brief statement (press release) of the facts of the case as known. This statement is simply read to the reporters over the telephone or in person. At this time the designated representative does not answer any questions, but should indicate when additional information will be available. This procedure should continue, with periodic updates, until the needed information is established. At this point, a final statement can be issued or the news media can be informed as to when they will have the opportunity to ask questions (i.e., have a press conference with the coroner or medical examiner). The press conference is held in much the same manner as the streetside interview, except it is usually not as frenzied.

In the case of a mass disaster, such as a commercial airplane crash, it has been suggested that one telephone line be designated solely for the news media. They can call this number 24 hours a day and will get a tape recording of information updated every so many hours. This frees up other telephone lines for calls from families, police, etc. and simultaneously provides updated information.

One caveat should be mentioned, for videotaped or live television interviews: you are responsible for your own appearance. Television news reporters are generally not permitted to stage the setting. At most, the video technician will adjust your seating angle, or remove a distracting object from your desk. But the neatness of your hair, the buttons on your blouse, and the zipper on your pants are your responsibility!

Lawyers/Courts (Expert Witness, Confidential Notes)

In the practice of the forensic pathologist, court proceedings are usually classified as litiginous (civil or criminal litigation) or evidentiary (inquests, grand jury testimony). Although the legal procedures and the ground rules differ, this system is generally conducted in an "adversary" fashion. Thus, while there are defined guidelines under which attorneys may defend or prosecute people or issues, they generally utilize the law to its fullest extent in an attempt to defend their strategy. The latter is of course potentially detrimental to the opposing side, and hence the phrase "adversary system of justice" has emerged. Court proceedings begin with no independent knowledge of a case. All facts are presented by oral testimony and the introduction of physical evidence. The ordinary or fact witness simply states what was observed to have happened. An expert witness is allowed to render opinions and draw certain conclusions. The term "expert" does not mean that the witness is the most knowledgeable person there is on a subject. It only signifies that the witness has sufficient expertise to allow for the expressions of an opinion.

The forensic pathologist is a neutral witness who simply provides opinions based on physical evidence, the circumstances of death, and background information. Hence, such opinions may be for or against the defense or the prosecution. It is crucial that expert witness testimony be strictly neutral and not slanted for the defense or for the prosecution or plaintiff. Expert witness testimony is only valuable insofar as that neutrality is preserved. And it makes no difference which side calls you to the witness stand. Opinions may be rendered in degrees of certainty. In criminal issues, the term "reasonable medical probability" is often utilized. This simply means that the witness is over 90% sure of his opinion. When the data base does not permit such surety, terms such as "consistent with," "possible and quite likely," etc. are perfectly acceptable responses to hypotheses by attorneys.

Some attorneys insist that the term "reasonable medical certainty" be used for a 90% or more degree of assurance, and "probability" be used for 50–90% certainty. This becomes a matter of semantics. But as one pathologist commented, if a fact is certain it does not matter whether it is reasonable or not! In either event, the terms allow for the fact that almost anything is "possible" and therefore various interpretations of fact exist.

Much ado is often made by attorneys as to whether or not the expert in forensic pathology is capable in subdivisions within his area of expertise (e.g., blood spatter, neuropathology, pediatric trauma, etc.). Since there are large overlaps of knowledge among experts in such fields and the forensic pathologist, there is nothing wrong with testimony from the forensic pathologist who is confident and experienced, especially in areas that rely on common sense. For example, there is no reason why the forensic pathologist cannot testify about coup and contrecoup brain trauma, or whether the round droplets of blood on the kitchen floor are consistent with drippings from a knife. For an attorney to suggest that only a neuropathologist or a blood spatter expert could testify about such matters is completely ludicrous. However, the witness should never go beyond his area of expertise. There is nothing wrong with saying "I don't know" or indicating that a cetain area of inquiry is in fact beyond your expertise. If asked what caliber bullet was removed from the body, a correct response might be "It appeared to be a medium-caliber projectile, but I don't know the exact caliber since I am not a firearms expert."

Although the vast majority of legal proceedings are conducted in a gentlemanly fashion, occasionally the medical examiner is the target of one of the attorneys. This is especially true in civil court, where large sums of money are at stake and the cause of death is a major issue. The pathologist should appreciate that there is usually nothing personal about such conduct and should remain calm, thereby answering the questions with careful consideration.

Pretrial Proceedings

After initiation of civil or criminal action, a subpoena *duces tecum* may be issued to all witnesses (medical or otherwise). The subpoena *duces tecum* is part of "discovery phase" of the pretrial proceedings. Thus, the attorneys are discovering the evidence and opinions for the forthcoming trial. A witness list is provided by each side, and hence each person on the list may be called or subpoenaed to appear before the opposing attorney and a court reporter so that a sworn statement may be recorded. The purpose of the deposition is to discover what knowledge (and opinion) a witness has of a case, and to "lock in" the testimony. Should the testimony at trial appear to differ from what was taken in a deposition, the attorney may "impeach" the witness to explain the apparent change in testimony.

Although these subpoenas are legally binding and do require attendance, if the day of the subpoena is not opportune the appointment can usually be changed to a mutually convenient time. Furthermore, a subpoena arriving with less than 3 days notice is usually considered inappropriate and may also be changed. Rarely, this action may require the help of your own attorney.

Prior to a deposition or other pretrial activity, the case file should be thoroughly reviewed and organized. Should a significant error suddenly appear in the autopsy report (e.g., right and left are reversed in a gunshot wound pathway), correct this neatly in ink, and initial and date the correction. *Never* erase or "white out" an error after the report is signed. At the appropriate time (e.g., beginning of a deposition), simply point out the error so the attorneys may alter their own copies.

The deposition is generally conducted according to a basic structure. The attorney will put forth his questions and the respondent (you) will then answer. Objections raised as to the form or appropriateness of a question are usually just formalities, and you are almost always allowed to answer the question. At the conclusion of the deposition, the court reporter will ask the witness if he or she cares to "read or waive." If one chooses to read the deposition, then the court reporter should provide the statement for correction. The deposition may not be significantly altered in content. However, significant factual errors, grammar, and spelling errors may be corrected. The deposition also provides the witness with a record of what was said during the proceedings. This is desirable for later preparation for court. Most witnesses, however, waive their rights to read the deposition because of time-pressure demands. Nevertheless, an uncorrected copy may be provided by either attorney prior to the courtroom proceedings. In controversial or complicated cases, it is worthwhile to read the deposition. Since many cases take months or years to reach the courtroom, it is wise to reexamine your previous statements and opinions.

Prior to or subsequent to the discovery deposition, conferences either via telephone or in person may be conducted with either attorney. Such meetings should be documented in the record as to person, place, time, and date. The pathologist is not obligated to discuss with the opposing attorney the content of these conferences if they indicate an attorney's theory or trial tactics. In fact, it would be ethically incorrect to do so unless so ordered by a judge. These meetings usually offer no problems when they are requested by the attorney who will call you as a witness in the trial (i.e., "his" witness). However, and unfortunately so, when the opposing attorney calls a meeting, there may be an objection. Even when there are no legal grounds for such objections, the adversary system tends to promote such protests. A "courtesy" phone call informing the other attorney that such a meeting will take place often reassures the attorneys of your neutrality. The fact is that the case may be discussed with any citizen, lawyers included. Also, it may be appropriate to remind an attorney that you are not "his witness"—your testimony will remain neutral whether he wishes to call you or is obligated to call you (because of the rules of evidence).

Day in Court

Prior to the court proceedings, a subpoena will request your attendance along with all notes, photographs, and other data to be brought before the court. The court date should be known well in advance and is legally binding. In addition, the court may extend the time frame of the subpoena (i.e., "a continuance") as it deems necessary. If the day of appearance is inconvenient for the expert witness, a better time can often be negotiated. Nevertheless, an appearance must be made and may sometimes interfere with vacation or educational leave plans. However, when the courts and attorneys are notified well in advance, other arrangements can generally be made. In addition, depending on the jurisdiction, the medical witness often need not wait in court all day to appear. Attorneys will generally notify you when your appearance is really necessary to avoid such waiting periods. Above all, communicate with the attorney and much time will be saved.

At some time early in the courtroom proceedings in criminal cases, the judge usually invokes the witness rule (or simply "the rule"). This signifies that the witnesses may not talk to one another regarding the case and may not sit in the courtroom as observers. They may only speak to the attorneys and the court. Such violation of this rule may result in contempt of court.

The first phase of questioning usually concerns the establishment of the expert's credentials. This usually entails a brief, or detailed, review of your *curriculum vitae*. The opposing attorney may stipulate to your qualifications to save time, or may do so because he or she may wish to subsequently diminish your testimony if it is potentially damaging to their case. Hence, the statement "the defense accepts the doctor as an expert in forensic pathology" may be flattering but also may be simply part of the defense's strategy.

The courtroom proceedings will then follow the usual rules of direct and cross examination, which may be followed by "redirect" and "recross." At the end of the session the witness may be "excused," meaning that he may not be called back to the witness stand. If the witness is not excused, he is still under oath and may be called again for subsequent testimony. If a court recess takes place during your testimony, then the case cannot be discussed with anyone, even with the attorneys.

The expert witness has the responsibility to answer the questions and the right to explain the answer. Hence, there is no requirement that an answer be simply "yes" or "no." If an attorney adamantly demands a "yes" or "no," simply answer and ask the judge if you may explain the answer. Furthermore, a witness should never fall into the trap of answering yes or no to a nebulous question or to a compound question (i.e., one part of the question true and the other part false). The attorney can always be asked to rephrase or simplify the question. One might simply say "I don't know," "I have no opinion," or "I don't understand the question." The latter usually stops the onslaught of even the most aggressive attorney, especially because the opposing attorney may strenuously object to further harassment of his witness.

Ideally, previous depositions should be reviewed prior to taking the witness stand. These statements may be used for impeachment during courtroom proceedings. If statements made during the deposition are at variance with your subsequent trial testimony opinion of the case, there is nothing wrong with changing your opinion based either on new information or simply a rethinking of the circumstances. Juries usually respect the doctor who will admit that he was wrong. On the other hand, if the attorney is simply taking the statement out of context or distorting the deposition, there is nothing wrong with politely telling the court about the distortion or the inappropriate extraction of the text. The witness may then explain the correct opinion or show how the statement was taken out of context by referring the attorney to previous lines in the deposition that he is holding in his hand. Remember, although you may answer "yes" to the question, "Doctor didn't you say on page 50, line 12 . . .," you may also explain your answer. Usually, when an attorney impeaches a medical examiner during a trial, it is because the question posed was different from that asked in the deposition.

During deposition or trial testimony, it is permissible and often necessary to refer to notes in the case file. This is done to obtain factual information about the case and also to document accurately conversations or other activities. It may be important to recall such activities, particularly if there is a discrepancy between your testimony and that of another witness, or if an attorney should insist you gave a different opinion on a prior occasion. The note should contain the case number, date, and time of the conversation and, of course, the person or persons with whom you were talking. The time of the note is as important as the date, especially if many conversations are conducted in the course of one day.

The precourt and courtroom proceedings should not be a fearful experience. The well-prepared witness is appreciated by the courts and attorneys. The most important thing, particularly for the novice witness, is to communicate with the attorneys beforehand to learn the ground rules. These will vary from one location to another, and also will depend on the type of proceeding (civil, criminal, military, evidentiary, etc.). In this jurisdiction, for example, depositions are frequent, whereas they are unusual in other areas.

A Few Helpful Hints for a Court Appearance

Before trial, review and organize the case file. Review your deposition if one was taken.

If you anticipate certain items from your case file will be introduced as evidence (e.g., photographs, diagrams), copy these ahead of time after marking the original with your initials in blue or red (any color except black). Insist on retaining all original documents. Generally, a copy of the original is all that is required, provided it reveals everything on the original photograph or document.

If necessary, review your *curriculum vitae* so that you may logically present your qualifications and experience to the court.

Answer all questions simply, directly, and in lay language. Remember you are really talking to a jury, a group of people of diverse backgrounds and education. You may, if necessary, answer in medical jargon "for the record," so long as you translate this for the jury. After all, one reason for the creation of a medical examiner is to explain complex medical concepts to a lay jury.

Never go beyond the scope of the question. If you do not understand a question, ask that it be clarified. If the question is compound, ask that it be rephrased (if the opposing attorney does not object to the format of the question).

Pause slightly before answering. This allows for the opposing attorney to raise an objection to a question on legal grounds.

Never go beyond your area of expertise. If you know the answer to a question beyond your scope (e.g., the bullet caliber), you may indicate that you know the answer, but that it is not your field, and let the court decide if you can answer. If you were told by someone else the caliber of the bullet, this is hearsay evidence, which generally is not permissible. When in doubt, let the court decide.

An *ad hominem* attack is an attack by an attorney on your credibility as a witness. This event is really quite unusual, despite perception. It most likely will occur during a deposition, since the attorney would not wish to alienate a jury, although it may occur in court if the factual case is particularly weak. Yelling or forceful language is usually designed to intimidate, and this is followed by interrupting your answers (and impeachment based on imagined discrepancies with your deposition if this occurs during trial). The only way to weather this storm is to stay in control: subdue your anger and fear, be objective, insist on completing the answers to the questions, never raise your voice, and stifle your contempt for the attorney and the system. Above all, be sure the jury thoroughly understands your answer, which means you must explain it over an interruption. A favorite tactic is to ask a question to elicit a "yes" or "no" answer and then immediately jump to another subject with another question. Again, stay in control: do not answer the next question until you have explained the "yes" or "no" answer. The attorney will typically retort that you answered the question, at which time you can respond by saying you had not completed your answer. Let the attorney get angry if he or she wishes, but at all times remain calm and professional.

Avoid acknowledging that an article or book is "authoritative" if at all possible. It is best to indicate that a certain text is a standard reference, but as with all such works, you may disagree with certain areas or statements based upon your knowledge or experience.

Use the terms "speculate" or "guess" to your advantage. You are not allowed to speculate. Hence, if you are pushed to render an answer that is not truly objective, use these terms. For example: "Doctor, do you know exactly how this wound was inflicted?" Answer: "No." "Does that mean you have no idea?" Answer: "Well, I could speculate on a number of possibilities." Then let the judge decide if you should speculate and opine which is the least likely or most likely possibility.

Above all, be neutral, informative, and professional. And don't let the problems of attorneys become your problems.

CHAPTER 2

The Medicolegal Autopsy

INTRODUCTION

This section outlines specific steps to be taken for the adequate documentation of unnatural deaths and the preservation of evidence. The interpretation of various injuries, blood concentrations of drugs, and the autopsy findings are not discussed. The reader is referred to any number of excellent texts and articles in the forensic literature that specifically deal with this aspect of forensic pathology.

The approach to the various categories of death presented here is based on the cumulative experience of this office, which has evolved into the procedures described. Although the overall approach is generally accepted among medical examiners, specific details may differ. It is expected that others may prefer different measurements, landmarks, or other details presented. This is perfectly acceptable, provided the documentation is adequate: the results should be understood by those who must deal with the work product for court or other purposes, and by those who may review the case file for purposes of consultation, interpretation, or research. The guidelines presented here will result in adequate documentation of medicolegal cases for even the pathologist inexperienced with such cases. The goal is twofold: first, that all necessary steps are taken so the case can be readily presented to other interested parties; second, that the documentation is sufficient for consultation with specialists in forensic pathology should there be a problem with the interpretation of a wound or with the autopsy findings.

Sudden unexpected death from natural disease is a fairly common event that forms a large percentage of the daily case load in any medical examiner jurisdiction. Since pathologists in general are basically trained in the delineation and interpretation of natural disease phenomena, this subject will not be addressed except for the sudden infant death syndrome (SIDS, crib death) and the chapter entitled No Cause of Death.

A chapter on nonfatal sexual assault is included, since coroners and medical examiners sometimes have the responsibility of examining these victims.

GENERAL COMMENTS ON TRAUMA VICTIMS

Ideally, the basic approach to a trauma fatality involves the following steps in sequence:

1. After the initial inprocessing procedure (fingerprints, photographs, etc.), examine the victim with the clothing on.
2. Remove the clothing and reexamine; photograph if indicated; inventory the clothing; allow to air dry and attach a property receipt if any items have evidentiary value.
3. Reexamine the body; X-ray and photograph if indicated.
4. Clean the body; photograph and diagram all injuries and distinctive scars, marks, and tattoos.
5. Take required skin biopsies (e.g., gunshot wounds, electrical burns, etc.).
6. Withdraw ocular fluid for toxicologic testing (usually alcohol).
7. Commence the autopsy.

Photographs of the body before it is cleaned usually have no value unless they depict items that will be obscured or lost by washing (e.g., gunpowder soot, glass fragments or paint chips in hair, "blowback" of blood and tissue on a hand, etc.).

Regional roentgenograms are routinely taken of all gunshot wounds (whether or not exit wounds are identified) and of all stab and puncture wounds. Full body X-rays (including the extremities) are routinely taken in the following instances: children below the age of 6 years (regardless of the apparent cause of death), explosion victims (bombing, industrial, or home), airplane crash victims, charred bodies, mummified bodies, and skeletonized or near-skeletonized remains. Bodies in moderate or advanced stages of putrefactive decomposition are not usually X-rayed, since the bloating tends to accentuate any penetrating injuries. Naturally, the finding of such an injury would require roentgenograms. Motor vehicle crash victims are also not routinely X-rayed, since the major fractures can be demonstrated (and photographed) during the autopsy.

The body diagram should record all significant external findings. External measurements are best made in inches, since most people (attorneys, jurors, etc.) have difficulty visualizing the metric system. Distances are always measured from the center of an injury to two convenient anatomic sites, which are, if possible, readily visualized by the lay person. The two sites provide for easy localizing coordinates. Typical landmarks easily visualized by a lay person include the external ear canal, top of the head, top of the shoulder (really, the acromion), nipple (for men and children), umbilicus, and the midline of the body. Other landmarks necessarily require anatomic terms and will probably have to be explained at a future date (e.g., the axillary lines, inguinal ligament, nipple line). Always keep in mind that a major historical reason for creating a medical examiner was to have somebody who would make complex medical terms and concepts easily understood by a lay jury.

Body diagrams made at the autopsy table generally have a myriad of shorthand notations and symbols, measurements, and sketches. Consequently they are usually unintelligible to everybody except the prosector. Therefore, when a case involves multiple enumerated injuries, it is advisable to make a clarification diagram to be attached to the autopsy report. This diagram merely indicates where the major injuries are and, in the case of gunshot wounds or stab wounds, the general direction. This clarification diagram is devoid of measurements and other notations that are included in the body of the autopsy report. Its purpose is simply to help the reader (including yourself!) to more easily visualize the major injuries described in the autopsy protocol.

For convenience, the headings in this section are divided into types of injuries. In reality, victims often have more than one type of injury, and therefore the autopsy report should be organized by the types of injuries observed.

GUNSHOT WOUNDS

In deaths resulting from firearms injuries, the purpose of the forensic autopsy is to preserve evidence and document those characteristics that will permit one to give reasonable answers to future questions. By the time the autopsy is completed, the pathologist should be able to provide the following information:

1. The pathway of the projectile;
2. A rough estimate as to the range of fire (if soot, stippling, or other features will permit this);
3. The amount and type of activity that would be possible after sustaining the injury;
4. The probable sequence of injuries, if this is possible;
5. The possible contribution of preexisting disease processes and, subsequently, the possible role of drugs or alcohol that may be detected.

Approach the gunshot wound case in a systematic and logical fashion. First, inspect and photograph the body with the clothing on. Remove the clothing and photograph all bullet holes on both sides of the garment. This often documents the presence of gunpowder and may help determine whether a wound is an entrance or an exit in some cases (Figs. 2.1 and 2.2). Reinspect the body and

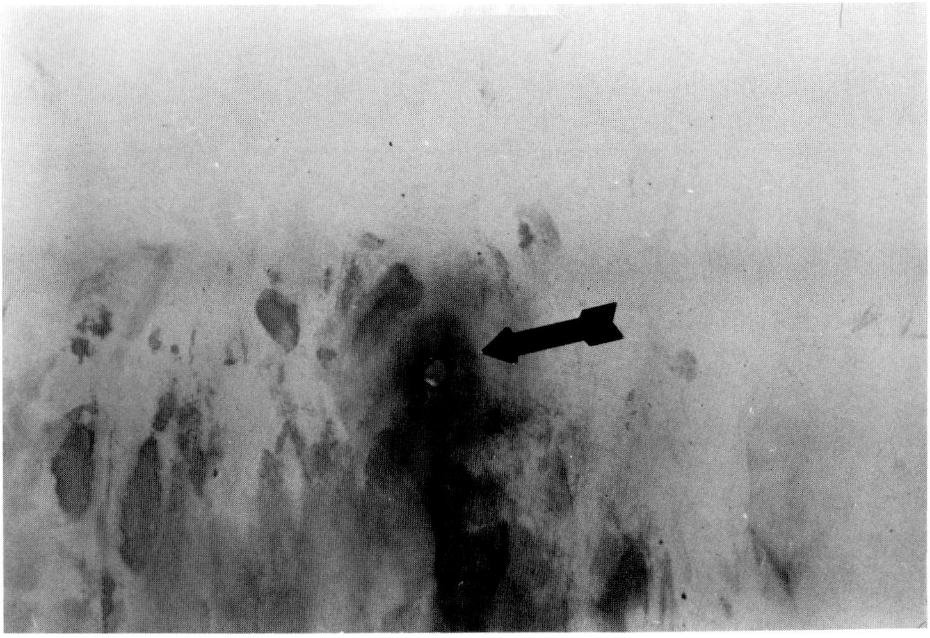

Figure 2.1 Contact gunshot wound with a large amount of gunpowder (arrow) around the defect in the clothing.

immediately photograph any wounds that have soot or other foreign material about them that could be removed by washing. Determine the areas to be radiographed. Clean the body and observe the characteristics of all gunshot wounds. Determine which are entrance wounds and which are exit wounds. These should tally with the number of projectiles detected radiographically. If they do not add up, reinspect the body, paying particular attention to areas covered by thick hair and to skin folds. Also consider the possibility of a slitlike exit wound (looking like a stab wound) that may have been missed, or a supported (shored) exit wound that may mimic an entrance wound. Reinspect the clothing. Reexamine the X-rays to be sure that the lateral edges of the chest, abdomen, shoulders, etc. are included. Finally, consider the rare possibility of a bullet embolus. If, after all this, things still do not add up correctly, one has no recourse but to proceed with the external documentation and a slow, careful autopsy to clarify the enigma.

Next, shave all hair from around the gunshot wounds (Fig. 2.3) and sketch the location of all wounds on a body diagram (Figs. 2.4 and 2.5). Always use the standard anatomic position, and localize the wounds by measurements from at least two fixed reference points. Wounds of the chest, abdomen, back, and buttocks should be localized by the distance from the top of the shoulder and the distance to the left or right of the midline. An optional third measurement

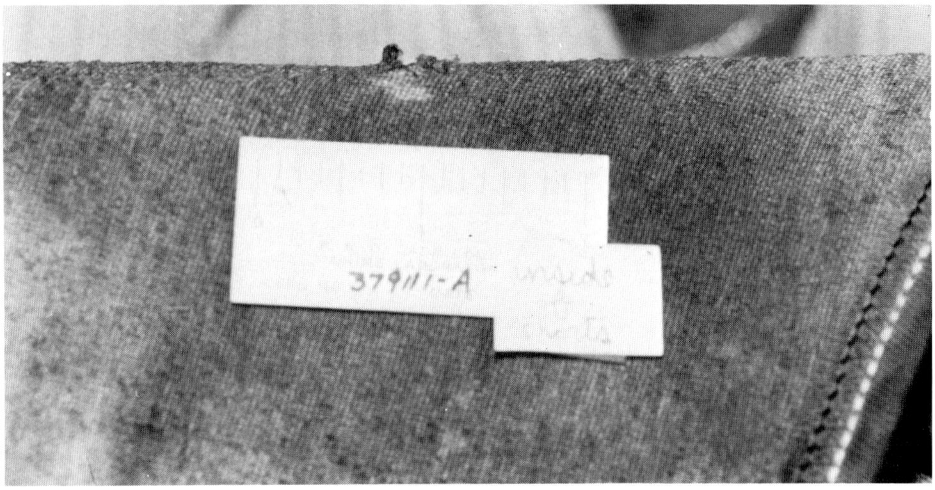

Figure 2.2 The deviation of clothing fibers may assist in determining whether a gunshot wound is an entrance or an exit wound in difficult cases.

is the distance from the top of the head or from a nearby anatomical structure (e.g., nipple, iliac crest, etc.). A gunshot wound of the head may easily derive coordinates from the external auditory canal or other suitable landmark, such as the occipital protuberance. The iliac crest is a suitable anatomic landmark for localizing wounds of the buttocks and pelvis. The axillary lines (anterior, pos-

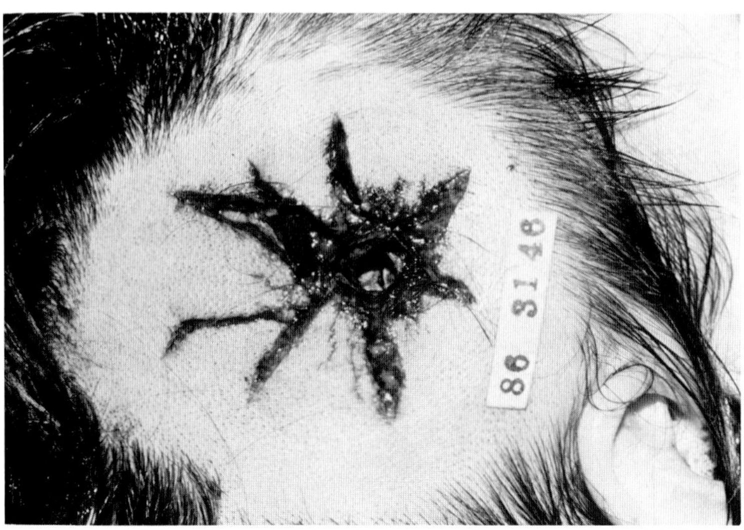

Figure 2.3 The hair has been shaved for a wide margin around this contact gunshot wound. This permits adequate inspection of the wound and its photographic documentation.

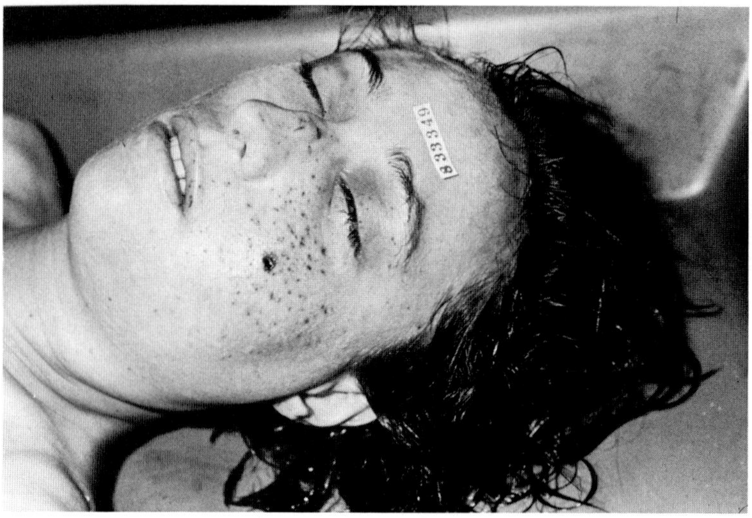

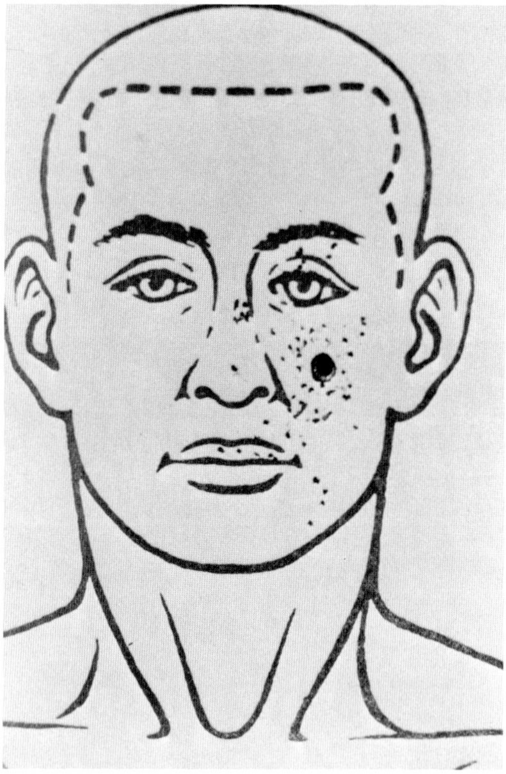

Figure 2.4 and 2.5 Injuries should be documented both photographically and schematically. The schematic depiction of this gunshot wound with powder stippling enhances what is visible on the photograph and provides backup documentation should the photograph be inadequate or lost. The diagram may also be useful for court testimony, particularly if the photograph is deemed inadmissible for any reason.

terior, and middle) are useful for the sides of the chest and flank. Also, distances from well-known locales, such as the antecubital and popliteal fossae, elbow, kneecap, etc., may be utilized. Ultimately, the body diagram will usually erase any confusion. Whatever sites are chosen as reference points, the purpose is to provide a clear indication as to the location of the wound and the direction of the projectile. Use common landmarks instead of esoteric medical terms, and measure in inches (or both centimeters and inches if you prefer). Also, the measurements are from the center of the gunshot wound perforation, not from the margin.

After localizing the wounds on the body diagram, note the size and shape of the perforation itself. Then record any characteristics of the wound margin (e.g., apparent gunpowder, abrasion ring, soot, stippling, etc.). If any abrasion or other characteristic is circumferentially uneven, then the unevenness can be described in terms of the location on the face of a clock (most prominent in the 1 o'clock position, most prominent in the 2 and 4 o'clock positions, etc.). Anatomical designations (anterior, posterior, medial, lateral) may also be utilized.

The vertical and horizontal spread of a gunpowder stippling pattern is important for estimating range of fire. The extent of stippling should be described not only as the distance from the center of the wound but also as a total area covered.

If gunpowder particles are loosely embedded in the skin, or even resting on its surface, samples may be removed for the firearms examiner. The gentle application of the tip of a scalpel can extract accessible particles. The latter can be placed into a fixative-free laboratory glass collection tube by tapping the scalpel against the tube's inner surface, thereby freeing the particle, or by simply placing the blade with particle directly into the collection tube. Loose powder may be picked up with clean adhesive tape.

When multiple bullet holes are clustered closely together (e.g., six bullet holes to the back of the head), it is often futile to describe each injury and trace its pathway. In that instance, describe the cluster, the area covered, the number of wounds, and the overall or average features of the wounds. Likewise, the internal injuries and projectile pathways must be considered and described together.

Graze-type gunshot wounds frequently have characteristics that indicate the direction of fire—e.g., the skin tags of a grazing gunshot wound point toward the muzzle of the gun (Fig. 2.6). Consequently, these wounds should be carefully sketched and photographed (Fig. 2.5). If the wound is on the scalp, shave a wide margin of hair from the wound margin and photograph the wound. Then have an assistant push the wound margins together and rephotograph the injury. This latter maneuver often clarifies the direction in which the skin tags point.

Commence the autopsy in the usual fashion, but be cognizant of projectile pathways and be alert for projectiles and projectile fragments. Dissect the areas immediately beneath all entrance wounds, and inspect for the presence of foreign particles (from a projectile or intermediary target). If the injury appears to

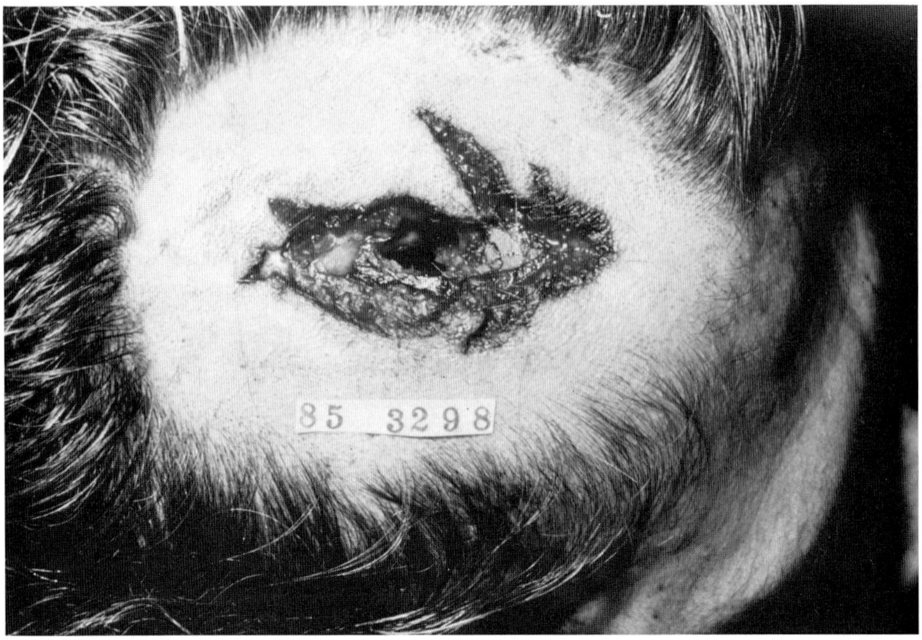

Figure 2.6 The skin tags produced by grazing-type gunshot wounds point toward the muzzle of the gun. In this case, therefore, the bullet traveled from the right to the left of the photograph.

be a contact or near contact wound, photograph the subcutaneous tissues to document the presence of a gas pocket, a pink discoloration from the gases, and gunpowder in the depths of the wound. Always collect a blood sample for potential serologic evaluation. The blood should be drawn by syringe and put into a tube without preservation (''red top tube''). Histologic sampling of entrance and exit gunshot wounds may be done for further documentation. However, bear in mind that a few particles of gunpowder may, on occasion, be microscopically visible in an exit gunshot wound.

Carefully note and photograph all bone defects created by the projectile. Skull and ribs are made of two layers of compact bone with a layer of cancellous bone in between. A projectile entering the bone generally leaves a circular ovoid defect with sharp margins (Fig. 2.7). As it pushes the disk of bone ahead, into and through the cancellous bone, it ''blows out'' the other side, creating a larger, more irregular defect, with beveled margins (Fig. 2.8). Hence, documenting these bony defects will clarify or confirm the direction of projectile travel.

Also photographically document all fractures that emanate from the entrance and exit defects of all gunshot wounds of the head. Since fracture lines do not cross, the finding of a fracture line that ends abruptly at a right angle with another fracture will also confirm which is exit and which is entrance: the fracture line from the exit wound is halted by the preexisting fracture line from the entrance defect (Fig. 2.9).

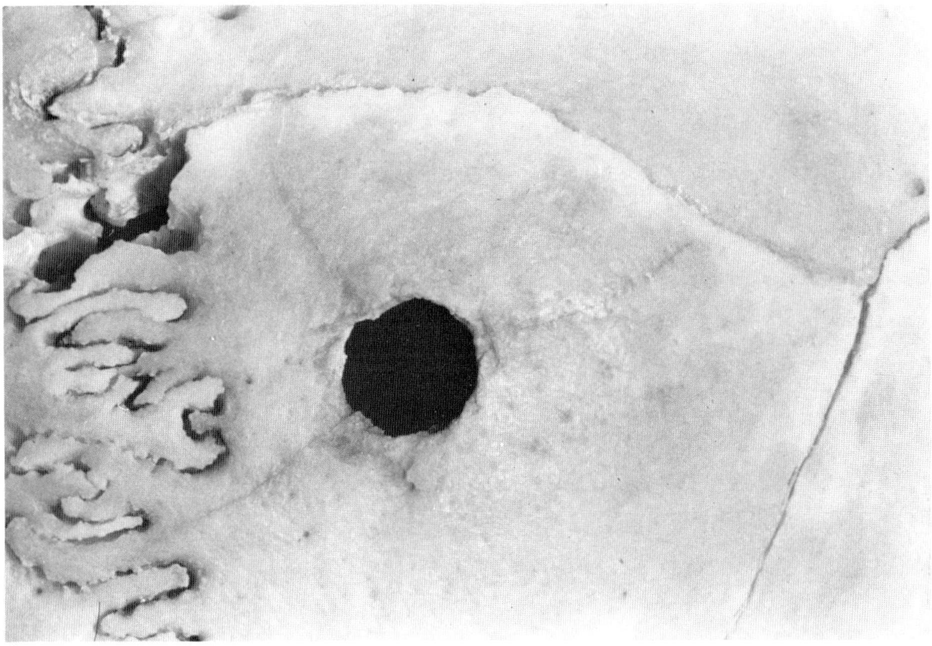

Figure 2.7 The circular, punched-out defect in the outer table of the skull (or other flat bone, such as rib) is typical for an entry site. The inner table will have a larger defect as bone is chipped away from the margin surrounding the defect. The inner table of the skull of an entrance gunshot wound, therefore, resembles the outer table of an exit gunshot wound (see Figure 2.8).

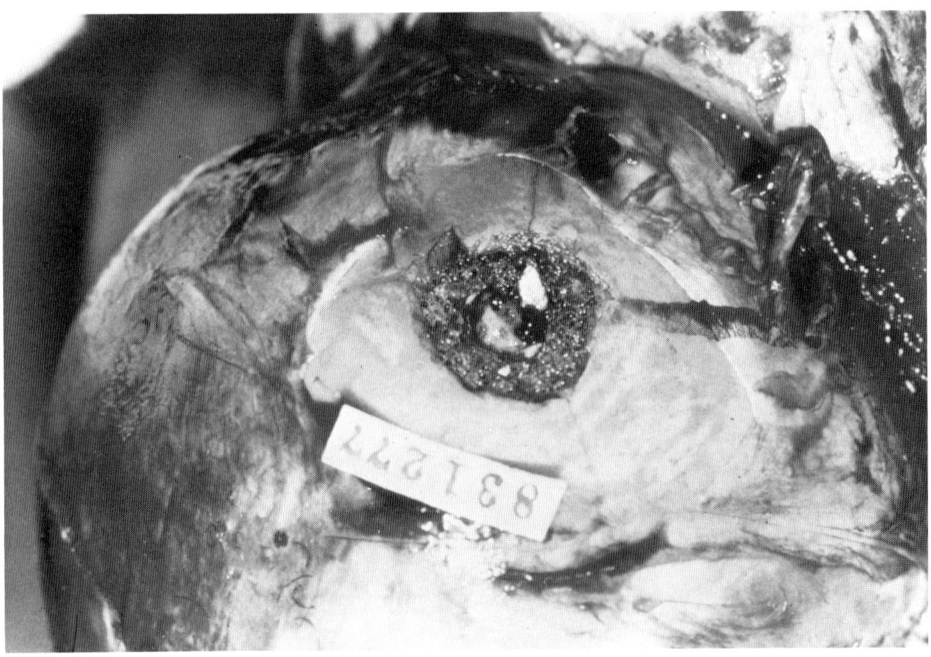

Figure 2.8 The outer table of the skull bearing an exit gunshot wound is typically beveled (i.e., the compact bone of the outer table around the central bullet hole has been chipped away). The inner table of this wound is a sharply defined defect, similar to the outer table of an entrance gunshot wound (see Fig. 2.7).The beveling features of gunshot wounds in bone confirm the direction of travel of the bullet.

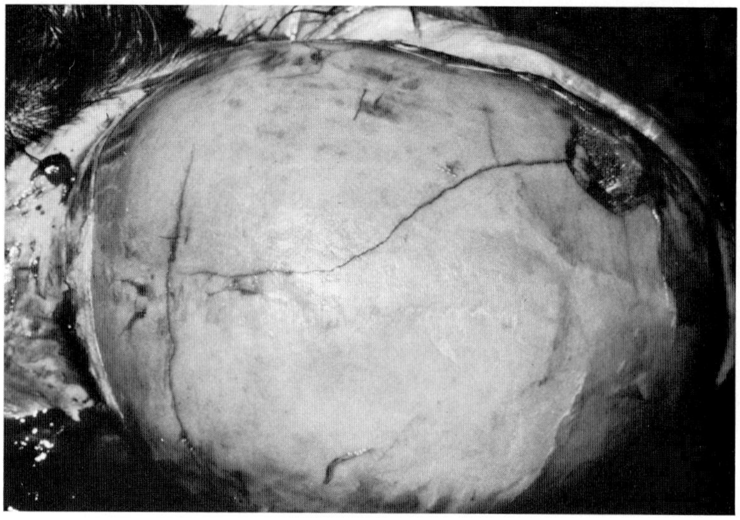

Figure 2.9 Fracture lines do not cross, since the energy of a developing fracture dissipates into an already existing fracture. In this case, the vertical fracture line (commencing at the top left from gunshot wound A) ends abruptly at the horizontal fracture line (which emanates from gunshot wound B to the right of the photograph). Consequently, it can be concluded that the horizontal fracture was there first, and therefore that gunshot wound B was inflicted before gunshot wound A.

Do not remove projectiles with metal instruments and do not place them in metal containers, since scratches will interfere with the lands and grooves so crucial to firearms identification procedures. Place the projectiles in plastic ice trays. If the projectile core and jacket have separated, keep them separate to prevent the core from marring or scratching the jacket, which has the rifling features (Fig. 2.10).

When the autopsy is completed and the projectiles are sorted out, they must be dried off and appropriately marked (except for shotshell pellets) at the base or nose with the case number and initials of the pathologist (if there is enough room). Use a vibrating engraving tool or a metal or diamond stylus (Fig. 2.11). If the projectile is severely deformed, simply do not mark it. Label a small envelope with the case accession number, the name of the victim (if known), what the envelope contains, the date, and your signature. Photograph the projectile(s) with their respective envelopes (Fig. 2.12), place the projectile(s) in the envelope, and seal it. Again, do not place more than one projectile in an envelope, and do not place a projectile core in the same envelope with the projectile jacket if they have separated. The envelope is then attached to a property receipt and given to the police. If the police are not there at the time, keep this evidence in a secured, locked area. The property receipt should read "brown envelope with projectile," to insure that the envelope and projectile stay together. Since you can't possibly put all the identifying information on the projectile, the envelope is proof that this was indeed the projectile you removed from that victim, and the photograph is backup proof.

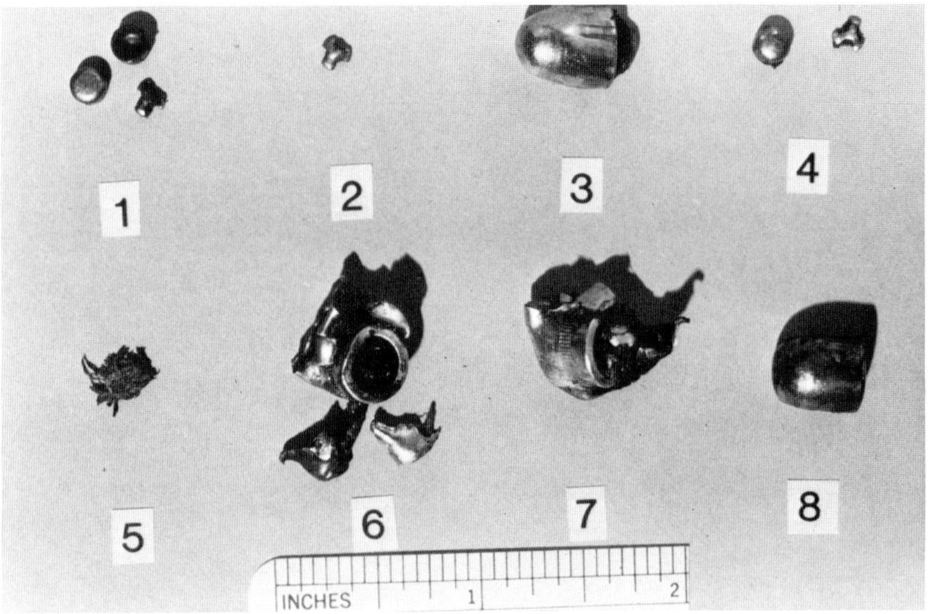

Figure 2.10 Multiple projectiles and projectile fragments must be kept separate. A plastic ice tray with numbered compartments is helpful during the autopsy. A composite photograph such as this may help solve any problems should the fragments become separated, or for court purposes. The photograph depicts the projectiles and fragments removed from a person shot with a machine gun loaded with exploding bullets.

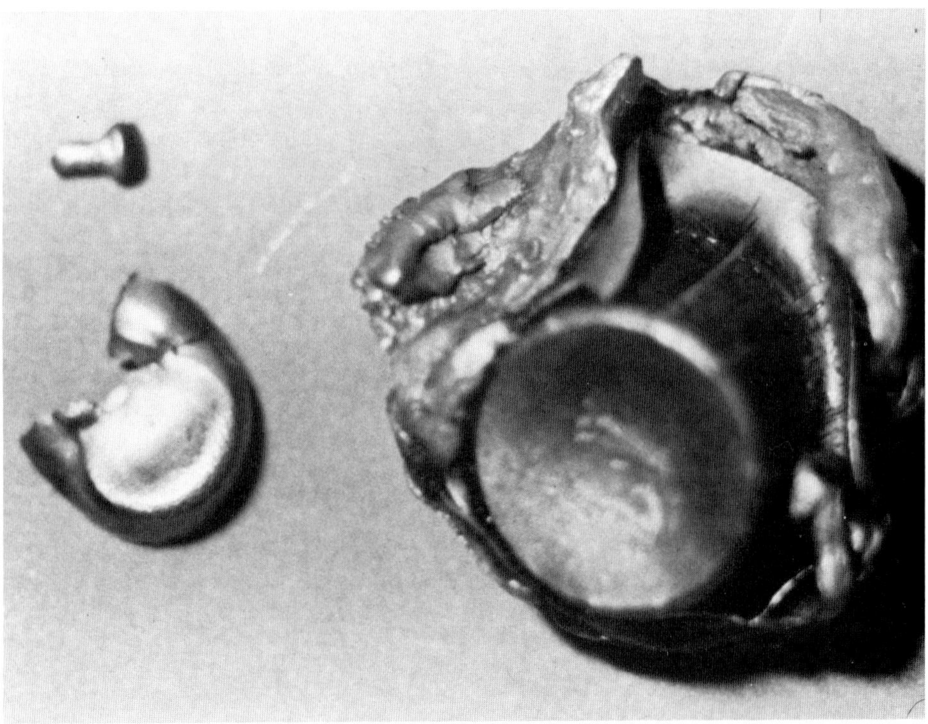

Figure 2.11 It is best to mark projectiles at the base with your initials or other identifiers. The nose or any other site not having rifling features may also be used. However, other sites (especially the nose) may have embedded trace evidence that may be destroyed by an engraving tool.

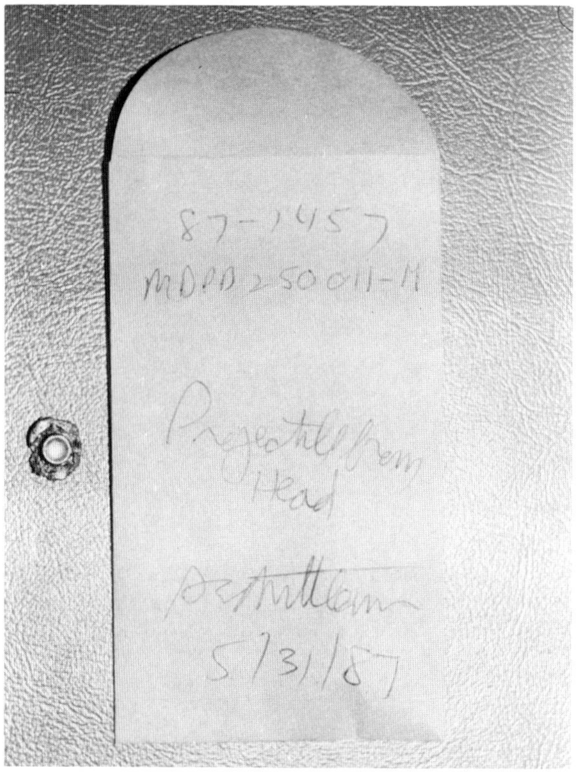

Figure 2.12 A photograph of the projectile alongside the marked evidence envelope facilitates courtroom verification of the individual projectile. It also identifies the medical examiner who handled the evidence.

In dictating the autopsy protocol, describe the entire gunshot wound from beginning to end, leaving the internal examination section to describe anything abnormal aside from the injuries. Begin with what the wound is (penetrating or perforating), where it is, the coordinates of the entrance wound, the characteristics of the entrance wound, the path through the body, and, finally, the exit wound coordinates and its features. The last sentence should summarize the overall pathway. Labeling entrance and exit wounds separately only causes confusion. If a person is shot five times, label the wounds "A" through "E" whether they are penetrating or perforating wounds. Describe the projectile in general terms only and never estimate caliber (since you are not a firearms examiner).

Example

Perforating gunshot wound to the head—The wound of entrance type is in the right temple, $\frac{1}{2}$ inch in front and $1\frac{3}{8}$ inches above the right external auditory canal. The wound itself is a $\frac{3}{16}$-inch circular perforation with a $\frac{1}{8}$-inch marginal abrasion containing a small amount of black foreign material that extends into the depths of the wound. At the 12 o'clock position, ¼ inch from the margin of the perforation, is a ⅛-inch by 3/16-inch, roughly rectangular abrasion from which extends a 1/16-inch-wide circular abrasion that surrounds the entire wound. Beneath the wound the temporalis muscle and extravasated blood have a slight red discoloration. The wound path continues towards the left with a sharply circumscribed circular defect of ¼ inch in the right temporal bone with prominent beveling on the endocranial surface. The wound extends into the right cerebral hemisphere, through the basal ganglia and the left cerebral hemisphere. Two fragments of medium-caliber copper jacketing are retrieved from the lateral horn of the left ventricle. The pathway continues through the skull of the right temporo-parietal region, resulting in a ¼-inch by 3/16-inch, sharply demarcated, ovoid endocranial defect with prominent ectocalvarial beveling. The external exit wound is a ⅜-inch by ¼-inch stellate defect without marginal abrasion. It is 1 inch behind and 2 inches above the left external auditory canal. The wound is associated with prominent cerebral edema, a diffuse extravasation of blood in the leptomeninges and subdural space, severe laceration and pulpification of the brain along the wound perforation, and scattered intracerebral hemorrhagic foci. The wound pathway is right to left, slightly upwards, and front to back.

Shotgun Wounds

Shotgun wounds may be described similarly to the usual handgun injuries. However, consideration of the scalloped borders created by the initial spreading of the pellets should be mentioned, since this gives some indication as to the range of fire (Fig. 2.13). When individual pellet wounds are encountered, the horizontal and vertical spread should be noted (Fig. 2.14). Also, look for any abrasions that may have come from the wadding of shotshell. The horizontal and vertical spreads of exit wounds from shotshell pellets are not particularly important to note, although the central focus of the cluster may be recorded. All large pellets (buckshot) must be retrieved during the autopsy to avoid allegations of a handgun's also being used. For small pellets (birdshot, etc.), only a sample of 10–20 need be retrieved. All wadding must also be recovered, since its presence is an indication of range of fire and also aids in the identification of the type of ammunition.

Summary

1. Examine and photograph wounds "as is."
2. Do entrance and exit wounds add up?
3. Examine clothing at sites of entrance and exit. Are the bullet holes consistent with your interpretations?
4. X-ray—whether or not there is an exit wound. Are the X-ray findings consistent with your interpretations?

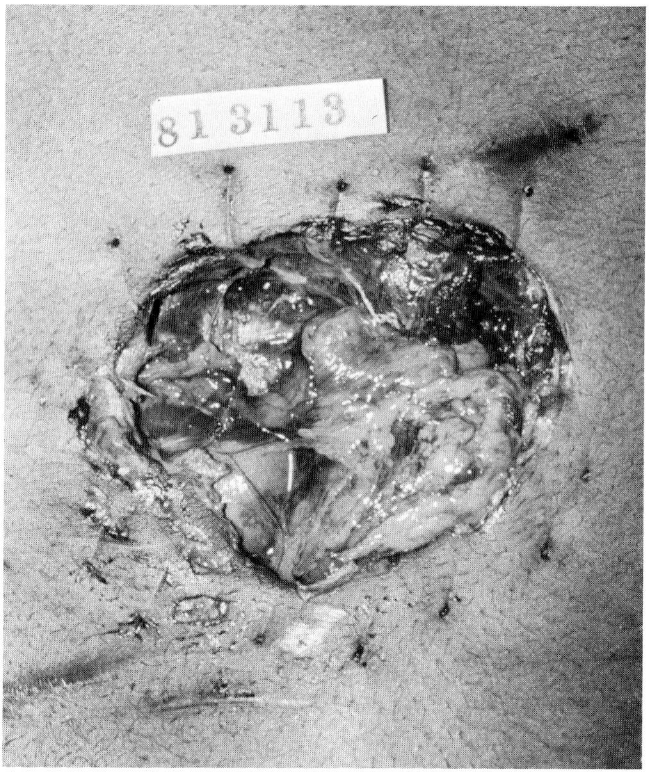

Figure 2.13 A shotgun entrance wound with scalloped margins and individual pellet wounds should be carefully photographed, diagrammed, and measured (like a gunshot wound) to help establish range of fire.

5. Photograph after cleaning and/or shaving area.
6. Make body diagram:
   a. localize entrance and exit wounds
   b. measure and characterize entrance and exit wounds.
7. Take histologic section of entrance and exit wound.
8. Perform autopsy:
   a. photograph any features that confirm entrance and exit wounds (e.g., beveling features of bone).
   b. obtain samples for toxicologic and serologic studies: ocular fluid, blood with and without fluoride preservation, urine, and any other samples depending on case.
   c. retain and photograph all foreign objects (or sampling of shotshell pellets). DO NOT REMOVE PROJECTILES OR PROJECTILE FRAGMENTS WITH METAL INSTRUMENTS. (These easily scratch the surface and obscure rifling features.)

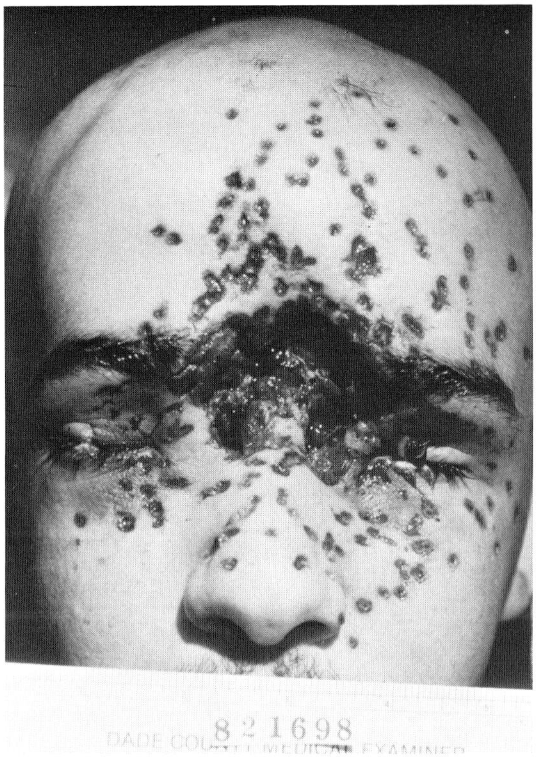

Figure 2.14 Measuring the vertical and horizontal spread of the shotshell pellet pattern (i.e., ignoring obvious stray pellets) helps to establish a range of fire.

9. Complete paperwork:
   a. mark and place projectiles in labeled envelopes.
   b. attach all evidence to property receipt and secure or give to police.
   c. complete toxicology request form; it is often best to hand the specimens to the laboratory personnel yourself, with a property receipt.

SHARP FORCE INJURIES

Sharp force injuries include stab wounds and incised wounds. In general, a stab wound is deeper than it is long, and an incised wound is longer than it is deep. Both are characterized by sharp margins, and the depths of the wound are devoid of tissue bridging (Fig. 2.15). All stab wounds must be X-rayed in the search for a possible knife tip that may have broken off upon striking underlying bone (Fig. 2.16). The knife tip is crucial evidence, since tool mark analysis may definitively link the fragment to the assailant's knife. The wounds should

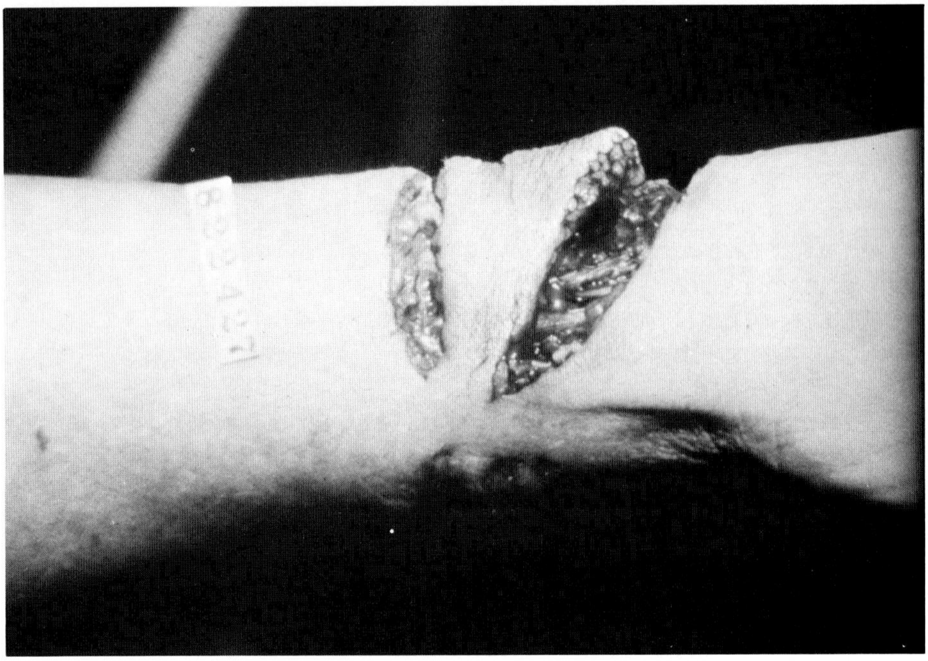

Figure 2.15 These incised wounds were inflicted by a boat propeller. Sharp force injuries have clean margins. Strands of tissue do not connect the wound margins (no tissue bridging).

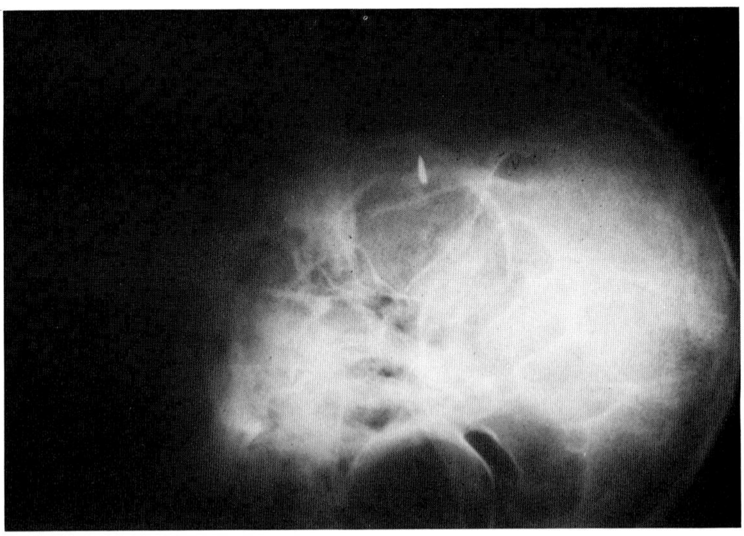

Figure 2.16 All stab wounds must be radiologically evaluated for foreign objects. In this case, a knife tip is seen in the radiograph. The knife tip, of crucial evidentiary value, would probably have been missed had the X-ray not been taken.

be described in terms of size, appearance, and location, as with gunshot wounds. Additionally, a notation must be made as to the orientation of the wound (vertical, in coronal plane, obliquely situated, etc.). Photograph "as is" with the edges gaping and then with the edges approximated with clear tape. Note any abrasions or other marks about the wound that may represent a hilt or quillon mark (Fig. 2.17). If present, these may be traced on a sheet of clear plastic (with the margins both gaping and approximated). Include the tracing in the case file. Be aware that the abrasion collars of sharp force injuries tend to dry out and may create artificially rounded contours. The dull side of a single-edge knife may create small tears at one end of the wound (Fig. 2.18), and this end may also have a rectangular appearance (Fig. 2.19). These features should be photographed and described.

The description of the wound pathway is similar to that used for gunshot wounds. However, it is important to realize that the depth of the wound does not usually imply the length of the weapon, because the body is compressible and also because the weapon may not have been completely inserted.

When the stab wound goes through cartilage, the cut surface must be saved in formalin for possible tool mark comparison with a suspect weapon (Fig. 2.20). This portion of cartilage is therefore the specimen with the most eviden-

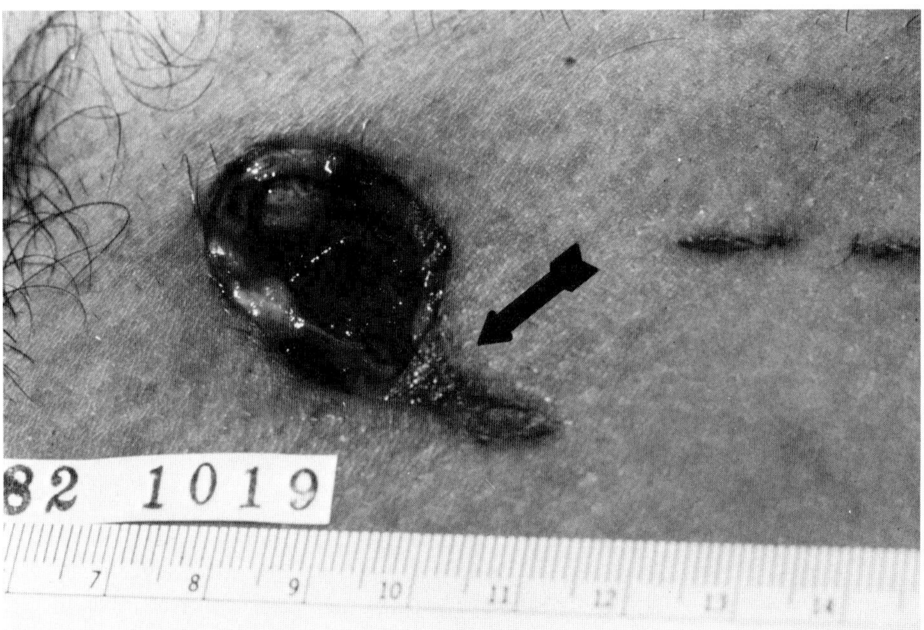

Figure 2.17 The abrasion extending from the 4 to the 6 o'clock position of the stab wound is a quillon or hilt mark, indicating the knife was thrust in as far as it would go.

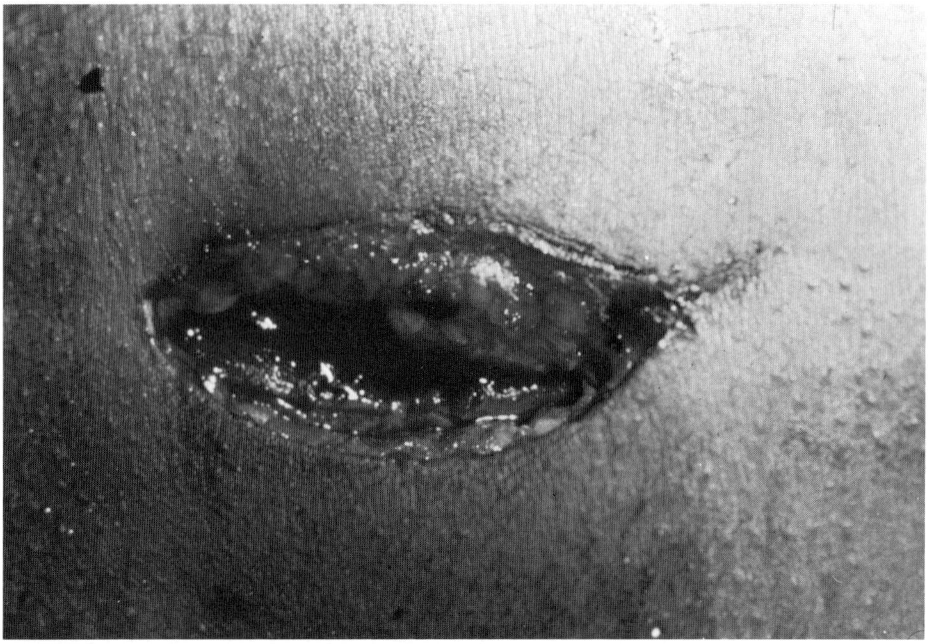

Figure 2.18 A small tear at one end of a stab wound is made by the dull edge of a knife as it is withdrawn.

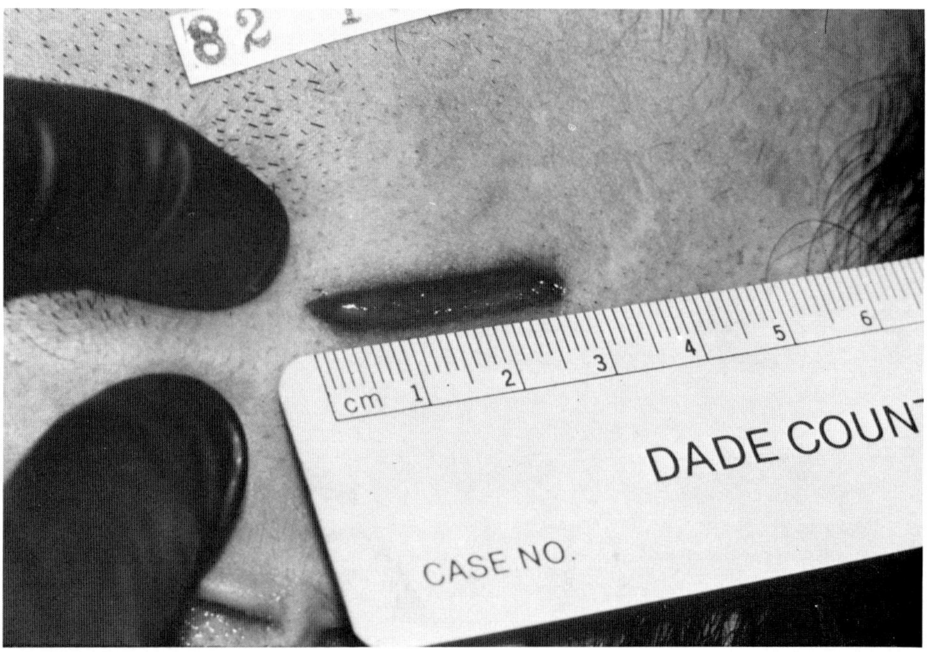

Figure 2.19 The rectangular end of a stab wound, best seen when the margins are pushed together, is made by the dull edge of a knife.

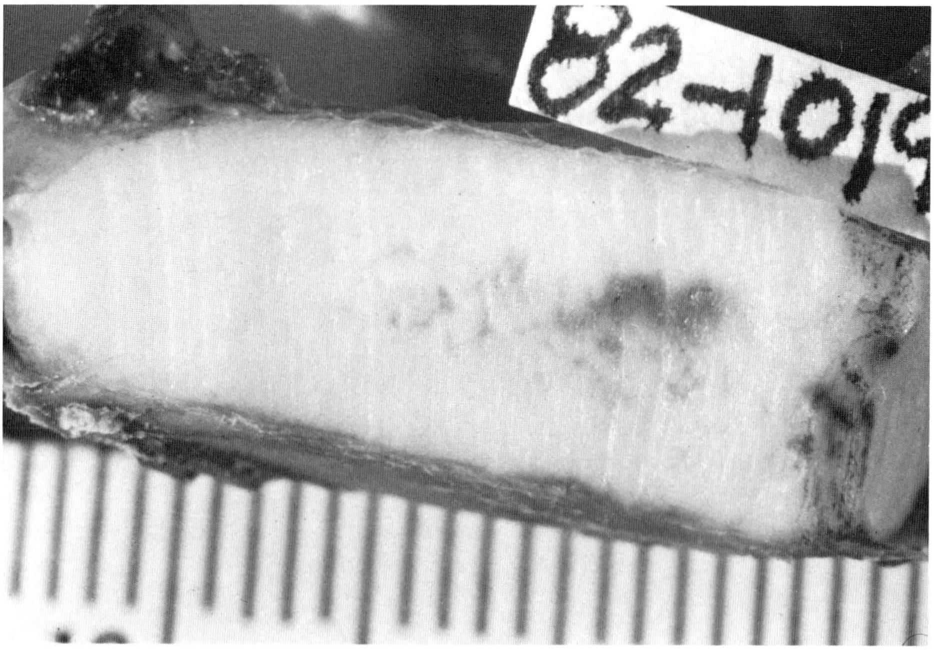

Figure 2.20 A knife plunged through cartiliage (in this case, a rib) may have striations on the cut surface. Tool mark techniques of the crime laboratory may reveal both class and individual characteristics to positively identify a knife as a murder weapon.

tiary potential. The entire stab wound in the cartilage should be extracted by cutting at least 1 inch away from the injury site and clearly marking with indelible ink the side cut by the pathologists's blade or saw. The markings (striations) on the cartilaginous surface should be photographed using macrophotography.

Keep in mind that a person with numerous stab wounds (''overkill'') may well be the victim of a sexually motivated assault. Consequently, the neck should be carefully examined for any marks suggestive of strangulation and a layerwise dissection of the neck may also be indicated. Obviously, pertinent swabs and other procedures (''rape kit'') to detect evidence of sexual assault should be done.

Victims with numerous stab wounds may be treated in much the same fashion as those with multiple gunshot wounds. That is, the wounds may be enumerated and described as clusters. For example: ''On the anterior aspect of the chest, 2 inches to the left of the neckline and 8 inches below the top of the left shoulder, is a cluster of 15 stab wounds covering a 6-inch area. The wounds average ⅜ inch long, they are vertically or slightly obliquely oriented, and the superior margins are rectangular when the wound margins are approximated. Their general direction . . . etc.''

Also, in cases of numerous stab wounds, make a tracing on plastic sheeting, which should also encompass easily identifiable anatomic landmarks (Fig.

2.21). A large sheet, which covers the entire chest and abdomen, for example, is an effective way to illustrate the location of the wounds to a jury. During the trial, the plastic sheet is placed against the body of a person similar in size or build to the victim. In this way, the wound pattern and distribution are easily visualized by the judge and jury.

Incised wounds are treated in much the same manner as stab wounds. However, one must be precise as to what was severed and not severed. This is crucial when the possible actions of the victim after sustaining such wounds are to be evaluated. Meticulous dissection is necessary, remembering that tendons, blood vessels, muscles, etc. will all retract and make the dissection difficult. If upper extremity tendons are severed, all must be accurately identified to conclude what function of the hands remained. In short, once the autopsy is completed, it is necessary to get out your favorite atlas of anatomy and slowly dissect. The same must be done for neck injuries and other situations where multiple structures have been severed.

On occasion an individual sustains a sharp force injury to a relatively minor vascular structure and dies without a large amount of external or internal blood loss. Usually the injured vessel is a small or medium-sized artery (e.g., posterior tibial), but it may be only a small vein (e.g., self-inflicted cuts of the

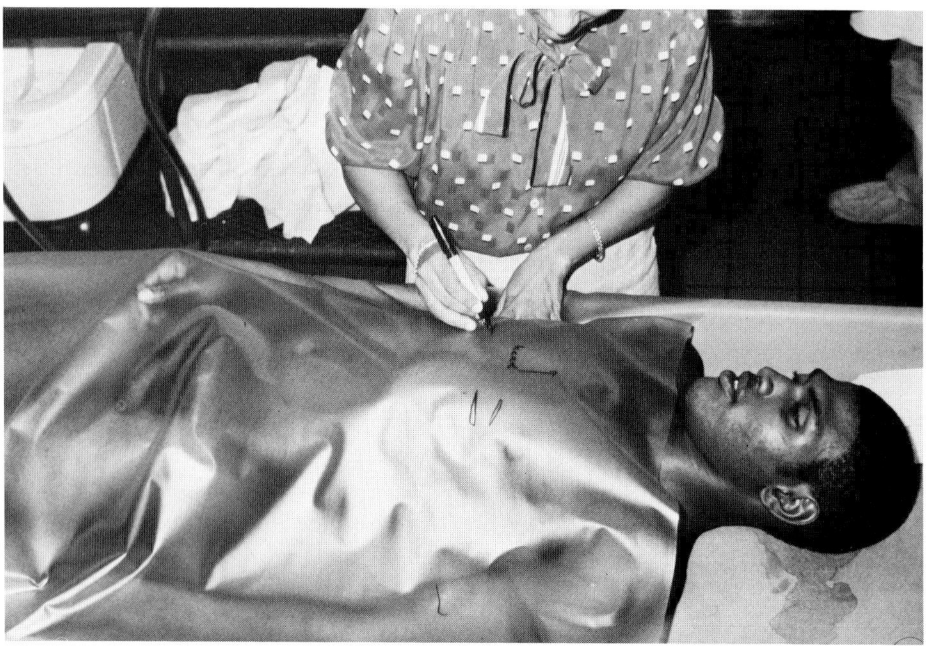

Figure 2.21 The location of multiple stab wounds is traced on a translucent sheet of plastic along with a few anatomic landmarks for orientation. This provides for additional documentation and serves as an excellent visual aid to a jury during trial testimony.

wrist). At the conclusion of the autopsy one therefore ponders the mechanism or even cause of death. It turns out that most of these individuals were severely intoxicated with alcohol when they received the injury. Some research suggests that alcohol intoxication (or even chronic alcoholism) renders a person more susceptible to hemorrhagic shock, possibly because the alcohol impairs peripheral vasoconstriction. In such cases, the cause of death is attributed to the vascular injury, and the acute alcoholic intoxication is listed as a contributory factor.

All victims of sharp force injury should have their hands and forearms specifically examined *and photographed* to document the presence or absence of defense wounds.

While performing the autopsy on a victim of sharp force injuries, anticipate the following questions: (1) "Which wounds would be nearly immediately lethal, potentially lethal, and relatively innocuous?" (2) "How much activity would be possible after receiving any one or a combination of the wounds?" (3) "In your opinion, how much pain and suffering would the victim have experienced?"

Summary

1. X-ray all involved areas.
2. Photograph "as is."
3. Photograph after cleaning.
4. Photograph after approximating the wound margins.
5. Photograph hands and forearms, even if there are no injuries (pertinent negative).
6. Trace wound on clear plastic (optional).
7. Make body diagram.
8. Perform autopsy:
   a. note depth of sound
   b. retrieve all foreign objects
   c. preserve and photograph all severed cartilage
   d. obtain toxicologic specimens
9. Perform special dissection as required.
10. Complete paperwork, etc., as with gunshot wounds.

BLUNT FORCE INJURIES

Blunt force injuries include contusions, abrasions, and lacerations. After adequate photography, their location, size, shape, and appearance should be noted. As with the sharp force injuries, it is usually not necessary to describe those characteristics which make each wound a true blunt force injury unless it is a crucial lesion (e.g., site of bludgeoning by baseball bat, patterned injury from a threaded steel bolt). However, if a laceration has smooth, nonabraded margins, specific mention should be made of underlying tissue bridging to distinguish it from a sharp force injury (Fig. 2.22). If this is the major injury, then it should also be photographed to demonstrate and document the tissue bridging.

Location of blunt trauma injuries may be described in terms of generalities, except when the lesions are of particular importance (e.g., multiple bludgeoning marks about the head). In those instances, the usual parameters of location may be utilized. Body diagrams are particularly useful for an overview of the wounds as well as for backup documentation in cases where blunt force injuries are numerous.

During the autopsy of victims of blunt trauma, the prosector must distinguish those injuries induced by attempts at cardiopulmonary resuscitation (CPR) from those caused by the traumatic event. Particularly troublesome are CPR-induced rib and sternal fractures, which may be associated with underlying injuries to anterior mediastinal tissues, and injuries to the hypopharynx and glottis from a difficult or traumatic endotracheal intubation. On rare occasions, CPR trauma to the liver may result in a totally iatrogenic hemoperitoneum.

Bludgeoning

With individuals who have been beaten to death, one must not only catalogue the wounds but also specifically consider four important factors:

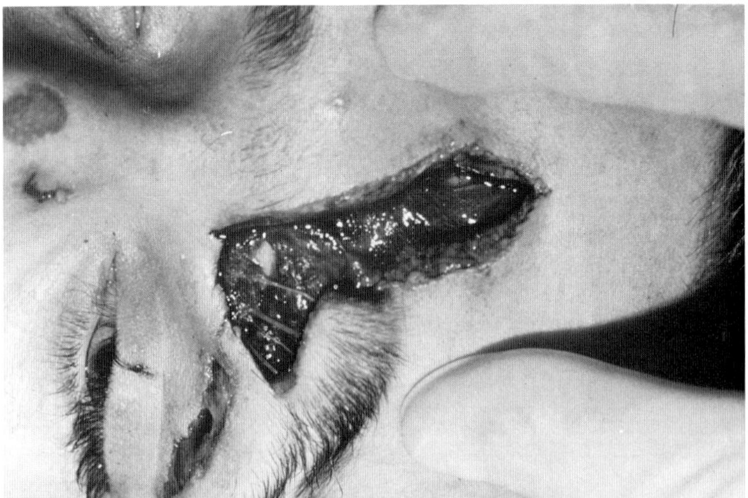

Figure 2.22 Tissue bridging in the depths of a laceration is characteristic of blunt force injury, and is not seen with sharp force injuries. Note the strands of tissue between the gaping margins of the laceration just below the eyebrow.

1. Are any of the wounds patterned injuries that suggest a particular instrument (e.g., threaded bolt, ax handle, hammer, signet ring, etc.)? Wounds of the scalp may well be associated with imprints of murder weapons (Fig. 2.23) and thus require additional photographic documentation (1:1 photographs with or without a ruler in place). Portions of injured bone should be removed and preserved when appropriate for subsequent comparison with suspect weapons (Fig. 2.24). Preservation in formalin or as dried cleaned bone will be suitable for future comparison studies. If a weapon is brought to the morgue for comparison with the wound, it is best that serologic sampling (of blood, hair, etc.) from the weapon be already completed. If this was not done, then remember that the weapon must not, in any way, touch the wound, since blood may be inadvertently transferred (Fig. 2.25). A note in the case file should indicate the absence (or presence) of contamination. Blood and hair standards must be obtained for comparisons with trace evidence on the suspect weapon.
2. Was the victim also strangled? Look for marks on the neck, petechiae of bulbar and palpebral conjunctivae, or other evidence of strangulation. When appropriate, a stepwise neck dissection should be performed, especially when there is also evidence of sexual assault.

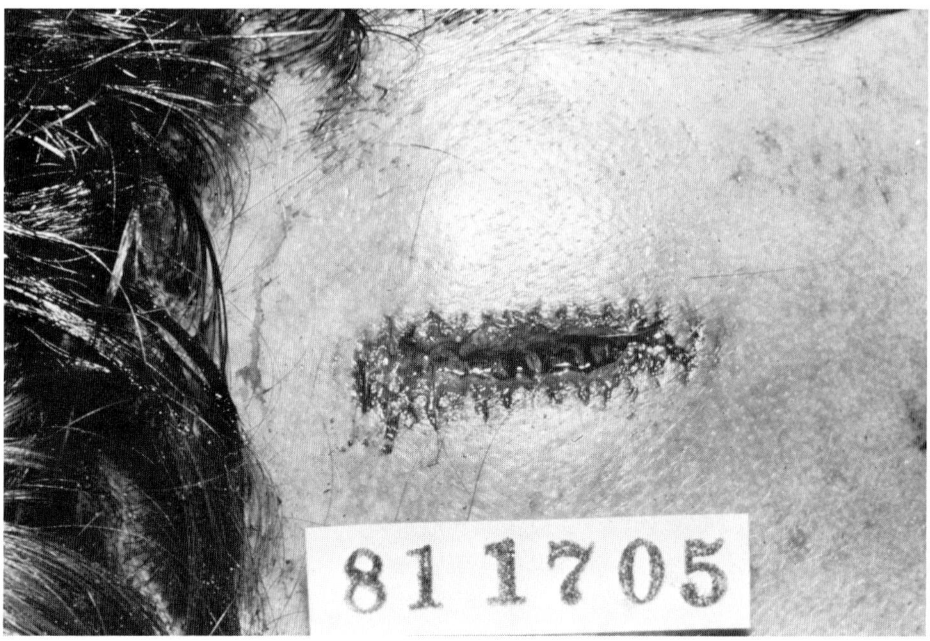

Figure 2.23 Patterned injuries from blunt trauma may offer clues as to a type of murder weapon. Consideration should be given to using techniques for bitemark evidence to properly document and preserve the pattern, in this case inflicted by a threaded steel bolt.

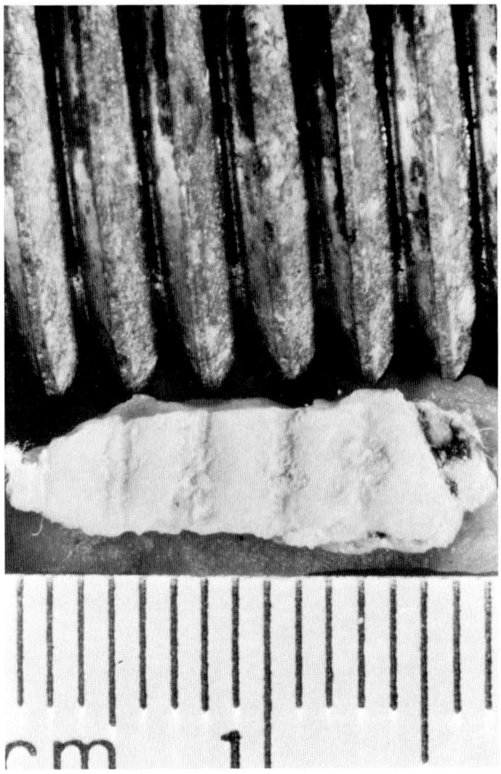

Figure 2.24 A blunt force injury may leave its imprint on underlying bone. The bone should be excised for later comparison to a suspect weapon (a threaded steel bolt in this case).

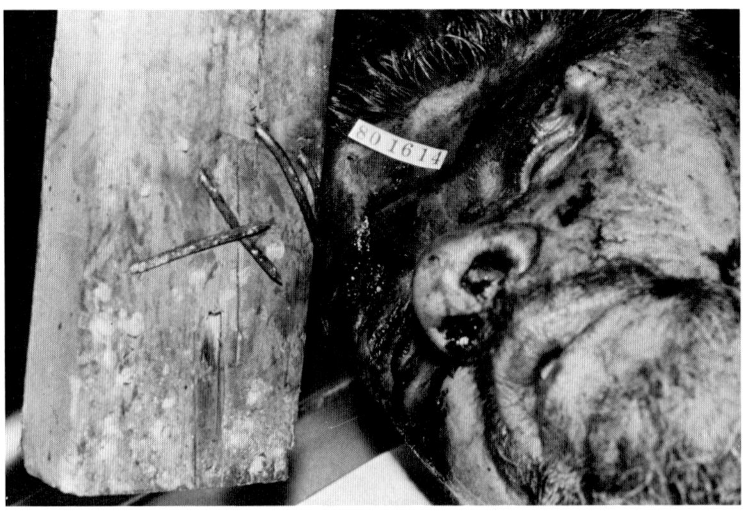

Figure 2.25 A suspect weapon should be compared to an injury at the time of autopsy whenever possible. However, if the weapon has not been processed for serologic and trace evidence (e.g., blood and hair), be sure not to touch the weapon to the victim. In this case, a 2 × 4-inch piece of wood is compared to a facial injury.

3. Are any wounds consistent with defense wounds? Look for trauma to the back of the hands and the ulnar surface of the forearms. A roentgenogram is useful for revealing fractures of the hands or forearms consistent with defensive-type injuries. Noteworthy is the "parry" fracture, a fracture of the ulna that is a defensive-type injury incurred during a bludgeoning (Fig. 2.26).
4. Is there a possibility that the bludgeoning was sexually motivated? This is a particularly important consideration in deaths occurring in all-male institutions (jails, schools, etc.).

Photographs of internal blunt force injuries are useful for documenting injury patterns such as a depressed skull fracture and coup-contrecoup injuries. These are also helpful in answering subsequent questions regarding the amount of force needed to inflict a particular injury and whether or not the wounds are consistent with a suspect weapon. These questions invariably arise during the course of criminal prosecution.

Any time injuries suggest uncontrolled rage (e.g., innumerable blows from a hammer or numerous stab wounds), one should specifically test for drugs that may release normal inhibitions (particularly alcohol) or precipitate hallucinations (phencyclidine, cocaine, LSD).

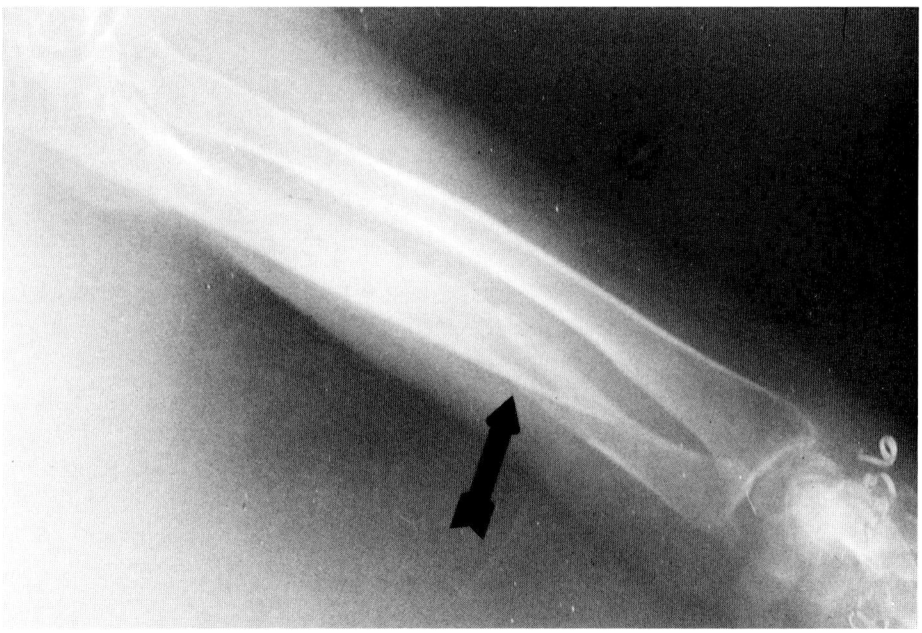

Figure 2.26 The fracture of the ulna (arrow) is consistent with a defensive injury (parry fracture) sustained during a bludgeoning. The X-ray not only detects and documents the injury, but is also useful during courtroom testimony.

Blunt head injury resulting in a subdural or epidural hematoma should be documented as to the location and the amount of blood accumulated. Histologic sections of the dura mater will aid in determining when the injury occurred. Also, if a scalp injury remains, a histologic section may further substantiate when an injury took place. Submit the subdural or epidural blood for drug and alcohol testing, since this may reflect the degree of intoxication when the injury was sustained (even hours or days earlier). Also be sure to differentiate a subdural or epidural ecchymosis (a thin, diffuse layer of blood) from the hematoma (a true, more-or-less localized accumulation of blood).

Sudden Death Following Minor Injuries

Sudden death during or shortly following the infliction of minor injuries is usually attributed to a disturbance of cardiac rhythm or to an intracranial hemorrhage. The typical scenario is that a person was engaged in a fight when blows were exchanged, and then suddenly collapsed. Postmortem examination reveals only minor trauma or no injuries at all. Details of the fight, along with the location of minor injuries (head or chest, or both) must then guide the subsequent autopsy procedure.

If the autopsy discloses natural heart disease (usually coronary artery disease), then the mechanism of death is most likely (within "reasonable medical probability") a dysrhythmia due to that disease. The entire scenario (not direct trauma) leads to the physiologic events that stressed a diseased heart beyond its capacity. The manner of death may therefore be homicide ("murder by heart attack"), depending on the circumstances and the temporal relationships. Knowing that the autopsy findings will invariably be scrutinized by others (including other pathologists), it is necessary to perform a detailed dissection of the heart with appropriate histologic sections. Literally, the heart should be "mapped out."

A direct blow to the chest may result in sudden death from commotio cordis. In this situation, the kinetic energy transmitted from the chest blow causes the heart to fibrillate, and the victim usually collapses within 15 sec after receiving the impact. The weapon may be a fist, baseball bat, or other similar object. The autopsy may reveal only minor external and/or internal contusions (Fig. 2.27), or there may be no visible signs of a blunt force injury. The heart may have a readily visible contusion, but usually it is grossly normal. Sometimes a hand lens will disclose a small contusion (extravasated blood) in the area of the atrioventricular node. Whether or not any bruises are visible, it is necessary to take multiple histologic sections of the cardiac conduction system, particularly the cardiac pacemakers.

Myocardial contusion following a blow to the chest (or from impacting on the steering column of an automobile) is usually observed after a period of survival. CPR may or may not have been initiated. The victim is often hospitalized for observations or because of other injuries, and then suddenly dies. In the majority of cases, the preponderance of evidence, including histologic sec-

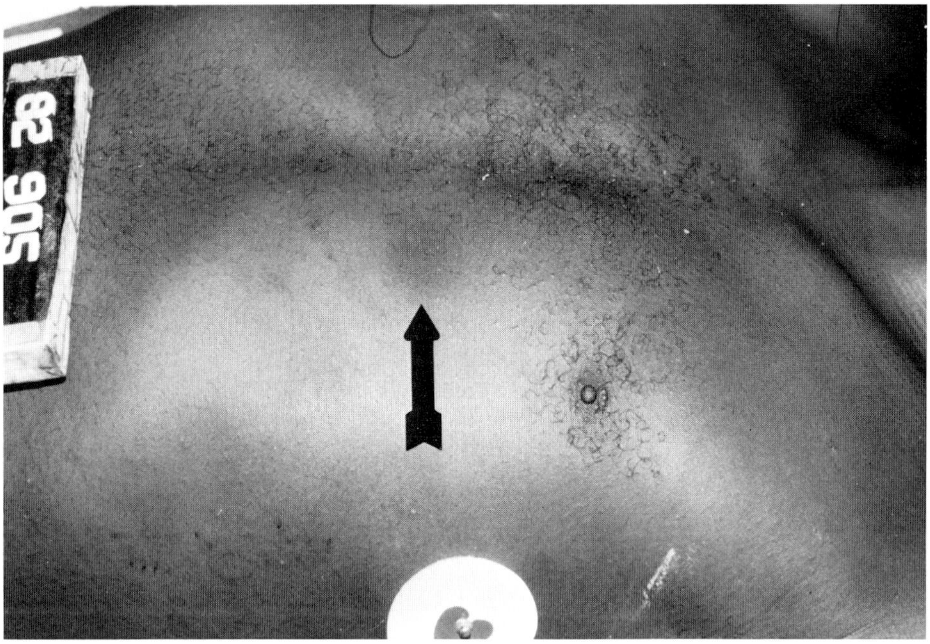

Figure 2.27 With sudden death due to commotio cordis, external evidence of trauma may be minimal or virtually nonexistent. In this case, the only visible injury is the contusion to the left side of the chest (arrow).

tions of the damaged area, will indicate the initiating event is the cause of the myocardial contusion. Anticipate the argument that the myocardial contusion was really the result of CPR attempts and not the injury itself.

Blows to the head that appear minor may be associated with intracranial hemorrhage from the rupture of an intracranial aneurysm or a lacerated vertebral artery. The former is the result of the event itself and therefore is treated in the same fashion as a "murder by heart attack." A laceration of the vertebral artery most often results from a blow to the chin or the mastoid area (Fig. 2.28). Again, there may or may not be any external evidence of injury. Death may have occurred during the inciting event or several hours later. History of the terminal event is therefore of paramount importance in determining whether or not postmortem cranial arteriography should be performed. It is best to anticipate the need for this procedure before beginning the autopsy. However, if an unsuspected subarachnoid hemorrhage is discovered upon removal of the calvarium, cranial arteriography may still be done. The point is that the actual anatomic defect must be identified: under no circumstances should one assume the spontaneous rupture of an intracranial aneurysm that "self-destructed and could therefore not be identified." This is crucial when there is a history of trauma.

In the situation of suspected subarachnoid hemorrhage from a lacerated vertebral artery, proceed with the organ evisceration as usual, leaving the neck

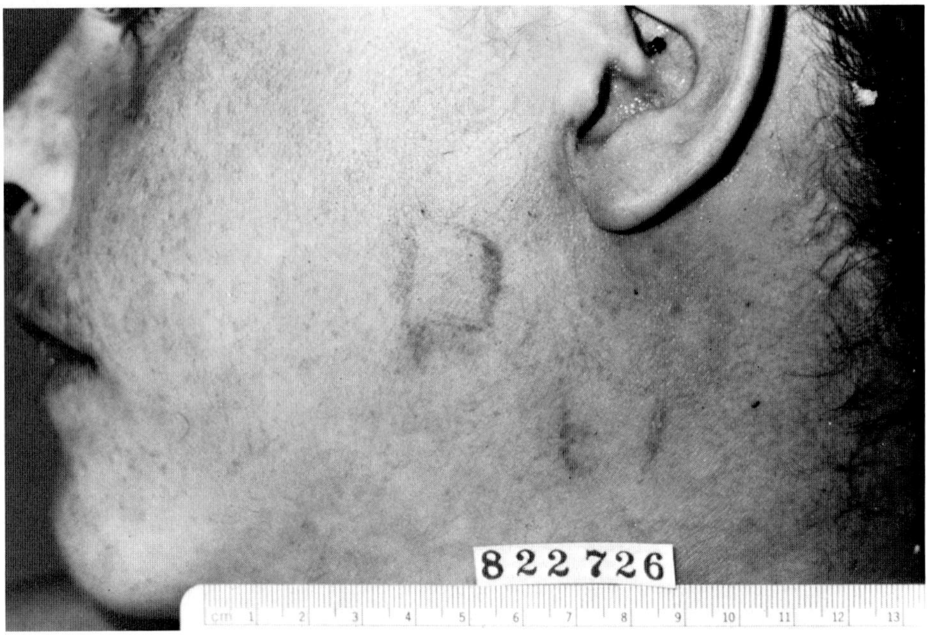

Figure 2.28 Fatal subarachnoid hemorrhage from the laceration of a vertebral artery may be associated with little external trauma. A faint ecchymosis is below the ear. The square abrasions were inflicted by a ring worn by the offender.

structures and the aortic arch intact. If the subarachnoid blood is discovered upon removing the calvarium, simply replace the calvarium and the reflected scalp to prevent undue disturbance of the brain. At this point obtain a lateral X-ray of the upper cervical vertebrae, since lacerations of the vertebral artery are often associated with a fracture of the transverse process of the atlas or axis. Also carefully examine the mandible (directly and radiologically) for a fracture, since this is also associated with a vertebral artery laceration. Next, isolate one vertebral artery near its origin, inject this with radiopaque dye, and X-ray the head and neck. Repeat this with the other vertebral artery. A lacerated vertebral artery demonstrated radiographically will necessitate a posterior neck dissection with ample photography and, usually, the removal of the atlas and axis. Removal of these vertebrae obviously provides additional problems for the undertaker. Hence, the insertion of a piece of wood (such as a thick dowel) will help stabilize the craniocervical area and be greatly appreciated by the undertaker.

Summary

1. Obtain appropriate X-rays for nonvehicular blunt force injuries:
   a. X-ray hands and forearms in cases of apparent homicide by bludgeoning.
   b. decide whether or not cranial arteriography may be needed.

2. Photograph "as is" and after cleaned:
   a. photograph and retrieve any foreign material of evidentiary value in wound or clothing.
   b. closeup photographs of any injuries suggesting a type of weapon, or patterned injury from a motor vehicle.
3. Note presence or absence of evidence of strangulation in apparent homicides.
4. In homicide victims (and deaths in jail), decide whether a rape kit should be obtained.
5. Describe and document injuries (make body diagram).
6. Perform autopsy, with careful consideration for toxicologic analysis. Be sure to save hair and blood samples for future comparison with a suspect weapon.
7. Complete paperwork as with gunshot wounds.

Motor Vehicle Fatalities

Motor vehicle fatalities should be approached to answer the following questions: (1) What caused the crash (human, mechanical, or environmental factors)? (2) What caused the injuries (correlation with crash kinematics)? (3) Is there any physical evidence to indicate whether the victim was the driver? (Survivors often point to the dead person as the driver, whether that was true or not.)

For the autopsy, two major considerations are required regarding the cause of the crash: toxicologic testing and the presence of any potentially lethal or incapacitating disease process such as coronary artery disease. The very minimum that should be tested for is carbon monoxide for all vehicle occupants, alcohol in both blood and ocular fluid of the victim, and drugs in the urine of the victim. Remember that low but significant levels of carbon monoxide may not impart a color change to the skin, blood, or tissues. Hence, test for carbon monoxide in all motor vehicle occupants.

Correlation of injuries with the crash events will be difficult or impossible unless detailed information is available concerning the vehicle, scene, precrash, crash, and postcrash events. In fact, some of these details may not surface for a year or more later. Consequently, all injuries must be thoroughly documented both diagrammatically and photographically, particularly when patterned injuries are identified.

The distribution and pattern of injuries may also aid in differentiating the driver from the passenger. If this is a possible issue, obtain scalp hair samples and blood samples for typing. Also carefully inspect the hair and the depths of wounds for foreign objects such as glass. Such evidence implicating a vehicle occupant as being a driver or a passenger may be important for insurance settlements, criminal prosecution, and civil litigation.

Some states now limit the amount of damages that may be recovered during civil litigation if the deceased was not wearing a seat belt. Therefore one can anticipate a question as to whether or not a seat belt would have prevented the death. Any injuries consistent with a seat belt injury should therefore be carefully documented.

In any pedestrian injury, sites of impact (broken legs, headlight imprints, etc.) should be measured from the heel. The location and nature of these wounds may provide some insight regarding the relative positions of the car and the victim, the type of vehicle involved, and whether or not the vehicle was braking at the moment of impact. Again, check the hair, clothing, and depths of wounds for the presence of foreign material (particularly glass fragments and paint chips) that could have been transferred from the impacting vehicle. This is most important in hit-and-run fatalities and when the driver was intoxicated with drugs or alcohol, since criminal charges will be likely. Hair and blood samples should also be taken for comparison with similar materials transferred from the victim to a suspect vehicle.

Radiographic documentation of fractures is usually not necessary in motor vehicle crash victims. In an aircraft crash, X-rays may give some clue as to the direction of impact forces and therefore should be taken.

Modify the autopsy report on motor vehicle crash victims so that all external evidence of injury is described first, and the internal injuries are described along with everything else in the Internal Examination section. This modification is not necessary in those instances where the only major injury is head trauma.

Jumps and Falls from Heights

Most falls from heights are suicidally motivated, fewer are the result of industrial accidents, and rarely are they of a homicidal nature. Because of the plethora of injuries, they are approached in much the same way as motor vehicle crash fatalities, including toxicologic testing. However, look for evidence of scraping alongside the building or injuries from impacting on protrusions from the building (such as a balcony or railings). Usually, a suicidal jumper will leap away from the building, whereas a person who falls accidentally will fall close to the building and attempt to grasp anything within reach. Always consider the possibility that the victim may have been murdered first and thrown from a balcony or rooftop to simulate a suicidal or accidental fall.

MECHANICAL ASPHYXIA

Death from any form of mechanical asphyxia may be difficult to identify, the signs of asphyxia often being nonspecific and subtle. In general, there are varying degrees of pulmonary and visceral congestion, pulmonary edema (most marked—with froth over the mouth—in drowning and mechanical chest compression), and petechiae of the pleura, epicardium, and conjunctivae. Petechiae may also be evident over the lips, face, and galea. Also check the lining membrane of the sphenoid sinus, it frequently has petechiae when they are obscured in the conjunctivae because of a prolonged postmortem state with the victim in a prone position.

Cardiopulmonary resuscitation may mimic, accentuate, or obliterate many of the subtle findings typical of an asphyxial mechanism of death. Hence, careful interpretation is necessary, especially when there is trauma to the neck induced by CPR (from jugular vein catheters and traumatic endotracheal intubation).

Always keep in mind the possibility of a postural (positional) asphyxia and smothering. In these cases, one may only find visceral and pulmonary congestion at autopsy. Also, one may find contact pallor about the nose and mouth and lividity of the remainder of the face. It becomes imperative to find out the exact position of the body when found and to interpret toxicologic results with care. In suspected smothering, always examine for contusions about the nose and mouth and inspect the frenulum for any blood or tears.

Drowning

In drowning victims, always make a specific note of the stomach contents (Fig. 2.29), the upper airway, and the sphenoid sinus for the presence of water, sand, or other foreign particles. On occasion, aspirated foreign material may be demonstrated histologically in the lung (Fig. 2.30). The petrous portions of the temporal bones are often hemorrhagic in drowning victims, and these should be specifically mentioned. The lungs may be relatively dry, markedly edematous (Fig. 2.31), or congested and edematous (particularly if the victim was intoxicated with alcohol at the time). In salt water immersions, the deep and peripheral gray matter of the brain is often accentuated (darker than normal), and this should also be mentioned. Pay particular attention to obtaining specimens for toxicologic analysis (especially alcohol). And forget the "drowning tests"; they are not reliable.

Food Aspiration

Regardless of the medical history, suspect accidental choking on food ("café coronary") in any adult who dies while eating, particularly when there is evidence of recent alcohol consumption. Persons with Parkinson's disease or other neurologic deficit that interferes with the motor function of eating (e.g., cerebrovascular disease) are also at risk to die in this fashion. If rescue attempts were undertaken, it is imperative that the rescuers' observations be obtained. The first thing rescue personnel do is clear the airway. Any obstructing foodstuff may be simply thrown aside during the rush of the event (in one case, the evidence—an obstructing piece of steak—was eaten by the pet dog!). If rescue

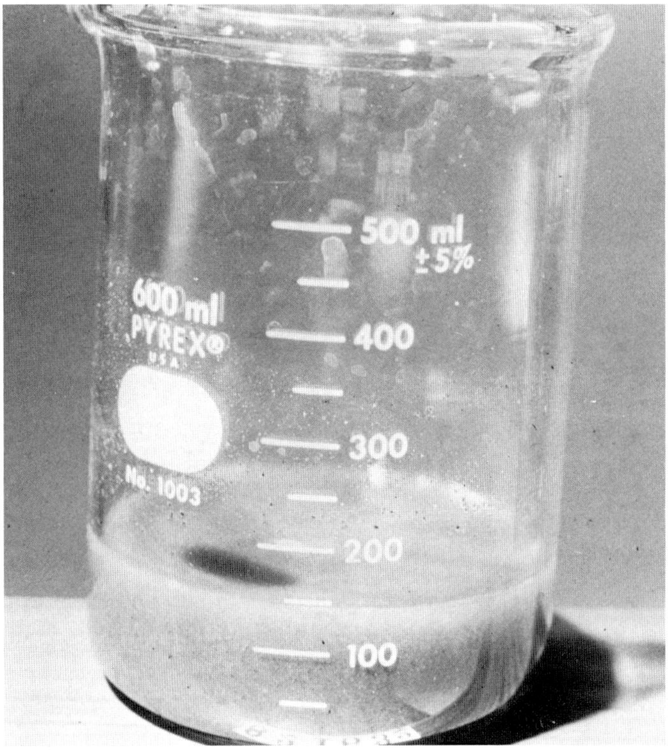

Figure 2.29 The stomach contents of drowning victims should be examined for foreign material. The murky water and silt from this murder victim provided evidence that drowning was the cause of death and that the death took place where the body was found.

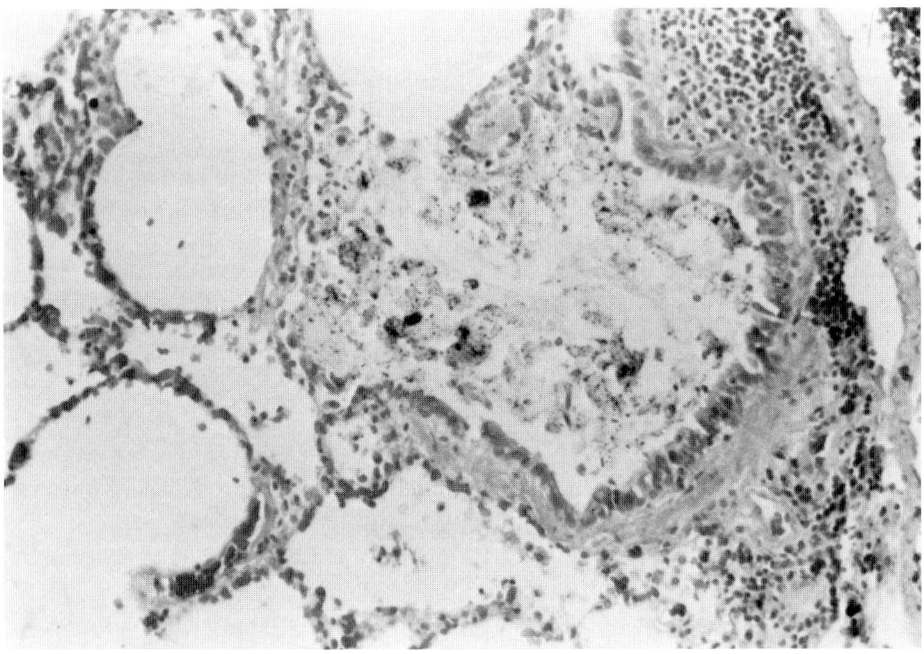

Figure 2.30 Histologic sections sometimes provide additional evidence of drowning. The amorphous black particles in the center are particles of mud aspirated during the drowning incident.

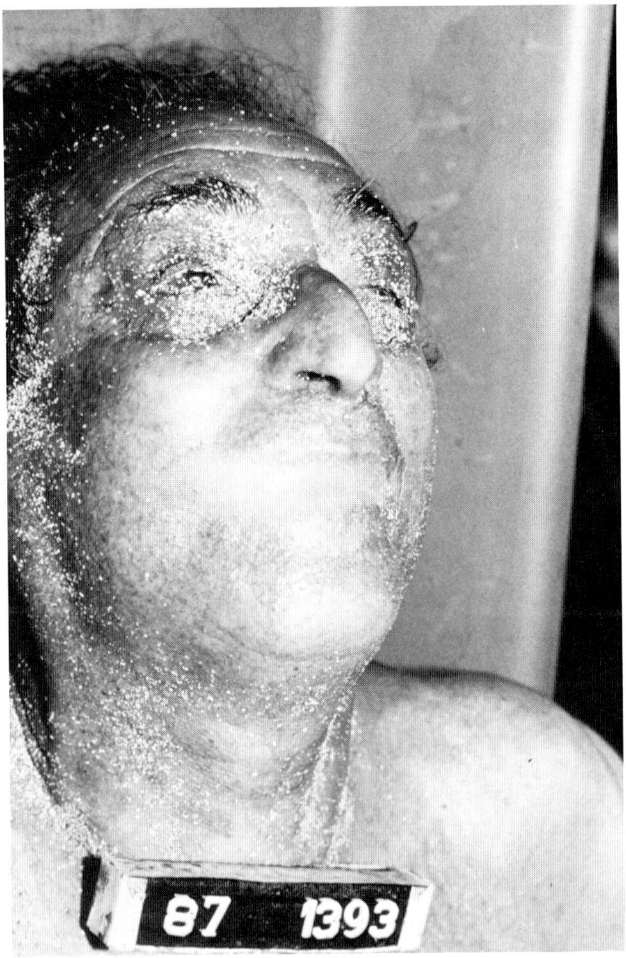

Figure 2.31 The white foam about the mouth is pulmonary edema fluid mixed with residual alveolar air. This is typical for nonintoxicated drowning victims. The face is covered with sand.

personnel did not find an airway obstruction, do not assume it was not there; solid chunks of food tend to get dislodged into the nasopharynx or forced into the trachea. Soft food (often the culprit among institutionalized adults) may get forced into the major bronchi and into the lungs from attempts at resuscitation. In children, suspect airway obstruction when they have been eating hot dogs or playing with smooth round objects such as marbles.

The autopsy will reveal the usual nonspecific signs of an asphyxial death. The obstructing foodstuff will be found in a supraglottic location or below. However, rescue efforts or even manipulation of the body may dislodge the obstruction to the posterior nasopharynx. In this location the object may be more easily palpated and extracted than visualized and photographed.

Do not confuse the café coronary with the aspiration of recently ingested food (vomitus). It is not uncommon for people to regurgitate food and aspirate the vomitus while succumbing to a natural disease process, especially if CPR is attempted. The two processes are usually quite easily distinguished. If there is doubt, then careful correlation of the autopsy findings with the scene and terminal events is mandatory.

Suicidal Hanging

When the body is said to have been found hanging, the ligature should be removed in such a way that the knot is left undisturbed. The ligature may be cut loose at any site along the loop, preferably the site directly opposite the knot, and the cut ends may then be taped together to recreate the original noose. The ligature should be retained as evidence, photographed, measured (thickness and length), described, and compared to any marks on the neck. The neck should be photographed to show the usual inverted V pattern (seen with most suicidal hangings) and a closeup of the ligature pattern (Fig. 2.32). If the ligature pattern does not have the expected inverted V configuration, then scene correlation (how the victim was actually found) is essential to exclude a homicidal death made to look like a suicide. It is best to obtain a picture of the ligature directly next to the pattern injury. Photographs should also be made of other evidence

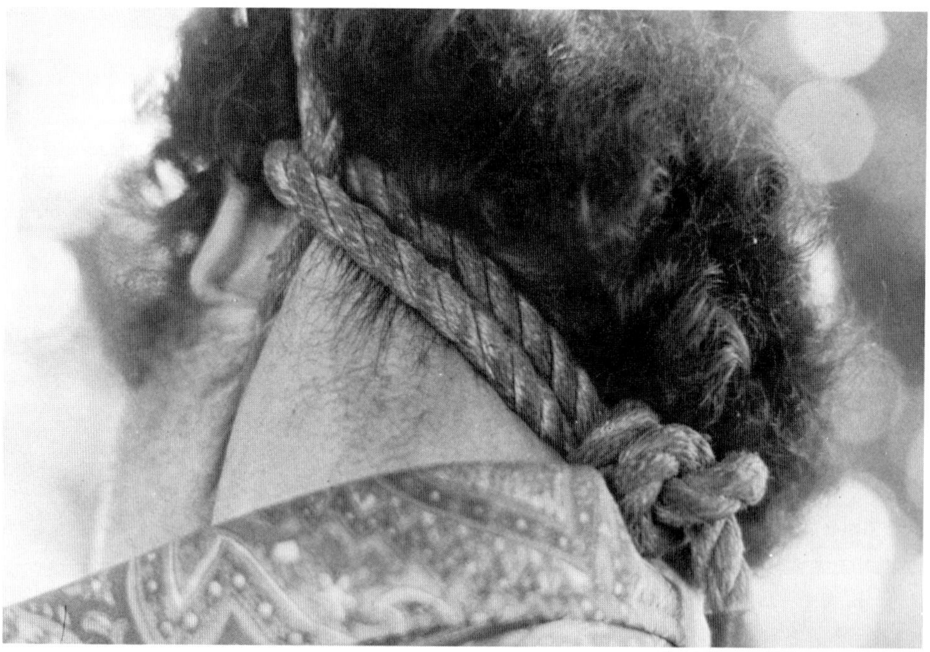

Figure 2.32 The apex of an inverted "V" abrasion on the neck of victims of suicidal hanging occurs at the point of suspension.

of injury, e.g., scalp lacerations sustained when the victim was cutdown, conjunctival petechiae, and Tardieu spots of the lower extremities, if present.

The neck should also be carefully scrutinized for linear abrasions and bruises inflicted by the victim in a last-minute attempt to remove the ligature. Of course, these could also have been inflicted by an assailant who then tried to make the death appear like a suicidal hanging.

During the autopsy one may encounter virtually no alterations of the neck structures in a suicidal hanging. Sometimes, however, a small amount of blood in the soft tissues may be found as well as fractures of the thyroid cornua or hyoid bone.

Accidental Hanging

In children, accidental hangings require a correlation of the autopsy findings with the scene of death. Each case is somewhat unique in that children become entangled in their environment in unusual ways: they get their heads caught in recliner chairs, in the slats of poorly designed cribs, or enmeshed with the strings of toys. Since the events and autopsy findings are so unique and varied, scene and autopsy correlation is paramount in establishing the preponderance of evidence for an accidental hanging.

Accidental hangings in adults generally fall into two categories: an unusual environmental incident or an autoerotic sexual asphyxia. The former occurs when the individual gets into a bizarre position from which they cannot be extricated, usually because of alcohol intoxication. An example is when a shirt collar gets caught on a wire fence during a drunken escapade. The uniqueness of such events requires close correlation with the scene, as it does in children.

Death from autoerotic sexual asphyxia is also fairly unusual, but a number of features occur with sufficient frequency to help establish the diagnosis. The death typically involves a white, middle-class male in his twenties or thirties. It is rare in females and blacks. Erotic literature and cross-dressing (transvestism) and a variety of forms of bondage are also common features. The ligature, usually a soft rope, is often padded so that the neck is protected. At the scene, a search should be undertaken to find evidence that this was a repetitive practice (e.g., finding a "kit" for this purpose, self-taken photographs or movies, numerous rope marks on a beam or tree branch, etc.). Also, evidence for seminal ejaculation should be sought. Historically, one must exclude overt suicidal tendencies. If bondage is evident, it must be established that it could have been done by the individual alone, and that an escape mechanism is present. The autopsy findings are typically nonspecific and are only those which suggest an asphyxial mechanism of death. However, despite the use of a ligature, externally the neck usually has no injuries or may have only minimal injuries. Toxicologic analysis is often negative, or it may reveal the presence of some recreational drugs (usually alcohol, cocaine, or narcotics).

Individuals who succumb to this type of sexual behavior do not overtly wish to die. Rather, their intent is to enhance sexual gratification. The enhancement is physical (hypoxia) and fantasy (skirting tragedy by the bondage and hanging, but overcoming the brush with death). Consequently, suicidal intent must be excluded by history and the scene of death, and it must be established that the bondage, if present, could have been done by the victim alone and that an escape mechanism is built in (Fig. 2.33). Historical or scene evidence of prior episodes of this behavior provides supportive evidence.

Death certification of these cases should not only satisfy vital statistics but also be sensitive to family members, who are usually shocked, dismayed, embarrassed, and bewildered. Even spouses are usually not aware of this practice and certainly never expected it of their husbands! It is our practice to certify the cause of death as simply ''hanging'' and the manner of death as accidental. For ''how the incident occurred,'' the sentence ''Deceased hanged self while experimenting'' is used.

One should also be aware that a common variant of this syndrome is to use an inhalant instead of a ligature. Common aerosol sprays (deodorants, lubricating agents for cooking) are most often used. A plastic bag may be used to inhale the fumes, or tissue paper stuffed into one end of a toilet tissue or paper towel insert may be saturated. These items will be found at the scene and are crucial in establishing the cause of death. When these agents are used, terminal vomit-

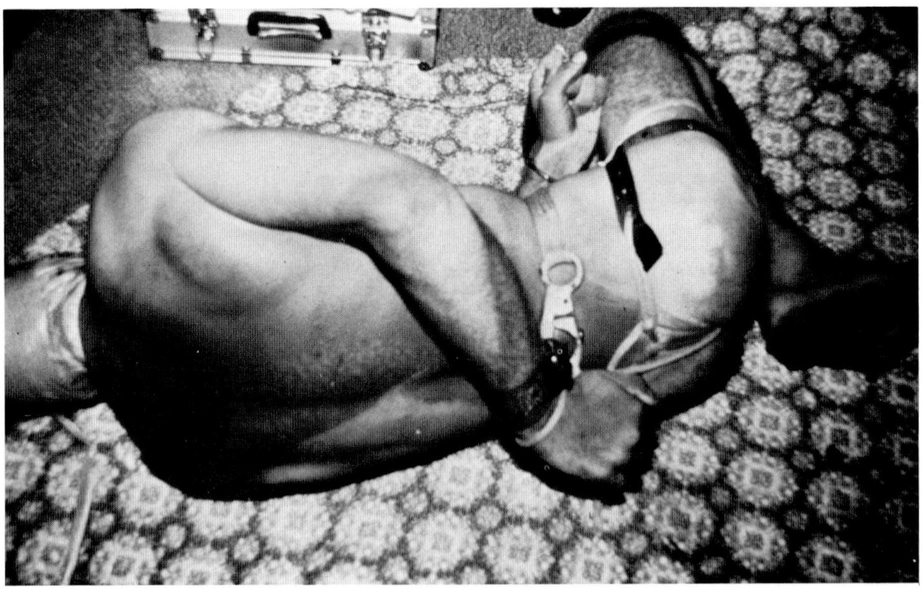

Figure 2.33 Fatal asphyxiation during an autoerotic event is often a bizarre scene. The asphyxia was produced by plastic wrapping over the mouth and a ligature. Bondage, but not cross-dressing, was evident at this scene. The escape mechanism proved to be the clip at the back; upon release, all the bindings relaxed.

ing with or without aspiration is common. If possible, the blood should be examined for fluorocarbons (e.g., freon), which are cardiotoxic.

Homicidal Strangulation

Intermittent hypoxia and an increase in cephalic venous pressure frequently result in numerous petechiae in the victim of manual or ligature strangulation, or when a person is strangled with a forearm or stick. These petechiae are most frequently found in the bulbar and palpebral conjunctivae, inner and outer surfaces of the lips, and the lining of the sphenoid sinus membrane. Also check for petechiae in the lingual and palatine tonsils.

In garroting, one or more prominent, horizontally oriented ligature marks are usually present. The ligature marks may have skip areas. Look for bruising (from a fist) on the back of the head and neck if the skip area is posterior. This results when the ligature is placed from behind the victim, who is then lifted up onto the back of the assailant, whose clenched fist supports the back of the victim's head and neck (Fig. 2.34).

In manual strangulation, abrasions may be few or very prominent and nu-

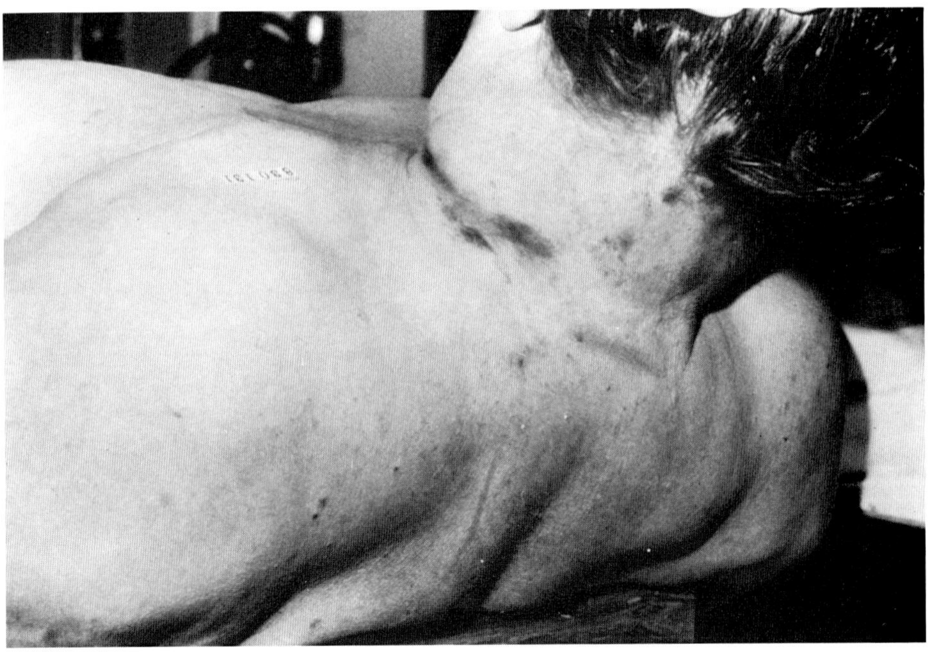

Figure 2.34 In a homicidal ligature strangulation, the neck abrasion is usually horizontal and the inverted "V" pattern typical of suicidal hanging is not present. The mark on the left side of the neck is the abrasion from the ligature. The contusions at the back of the neck are from a fist. The ligature was placed around the victim's neck from behind and twisted posteriorly, and the victim was then lifted onto the shoulder or back of the assailant. The fist formed a fulcrum at the back of the neck.

merous. However, if a body is removed from water (lake, ocean, or bathtub), do not commence the postmortem examination (except for evidence collection in a suspected sexual assault) until the body is thoroughly dry. This is usually accomplished by overnight storage. The reason for being sure the body is dry is that ABRASIONS CANNOT BE VISUALIZED IF THEY ARE WET (Fig. 2.35). Abrasions must dehydrate before they are visible (actually, as the body surface dries, the abrasions will become visible in a fashion resembling a developing photograph).

Before proceeding with the autopsy, consult with the police as to whether they need a workup for sexual assault, or fingernail scrapings and clippings for trace evidence (possibility of hair, blood, or skin of the assailant).

Layerwise Neck Dissection

This procedure is mandatory for confirming and establishing (or refuting) a homicidal strangulation. Prior to a neck dissection, the thoracic, abdominal, and cranial contents should be eviscerated so that the body is drained of blood. This will prevent any artifactual extravasation of blood into the soft tissues of the neck.

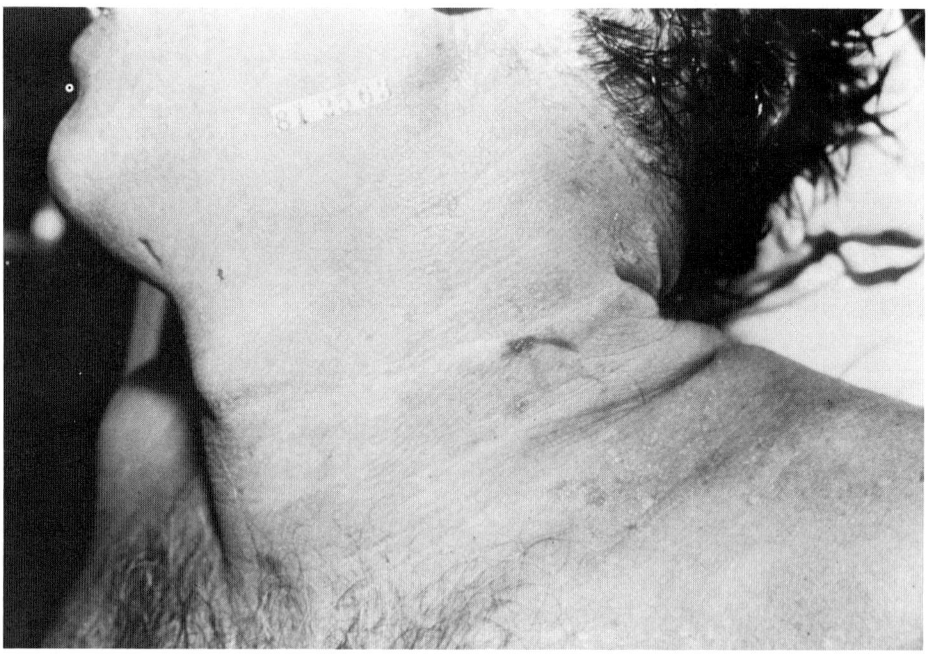

Figure 2.35 This man was found dead in a bathtub full of water. At the scene, no neck abrasions or other evidence of trauma was seen. The next morning, the neck abrasions were evident. They strongly suggest the possibility of manual strangulation, which, in fact, was the cause of death. ABRASIONS ARE NOT VISIBLE IF THEY ARE WET.

A sharp scalpel blade (which should be periodically changed during the dissection) is the only necessary tool. Use the tip of the knife to dissect, rather than the blade itself. The skin, subcutis, and adherent platysma are reflected as one layer, using the left hand (not a forceps) to retract the flap. Stay close to the skin flap rather than the muscle. The skin flap is reflected above the thyroid cartilage. This is facilitated by using relaxing incisions, i.e., the interacromion skin incision is extended slightly towards both shoulders.

Next, the muscles are dissected. It is best to reflect the neck muscles on both sides simultaneously rather than completing one side and then doing the other. This way, one can visually compare and evaluate any smaller hemorrhagic foci, using the side that is uninvolved as a sort of negative control. Each step of the dissection is photographed, even if no injury is apparent. Incise the sternal and clavicular attachments and the medial and lateral bellies of the sternocleidomastoid muscles and reflect them upwards. The next layer to be reflected is the delicate omohyoid muscle, followed by the "strap muscles": sternohyoid, sternothyroid (medial and lateral), and thyrohyoid (Fig. 2.36). The layers are easy

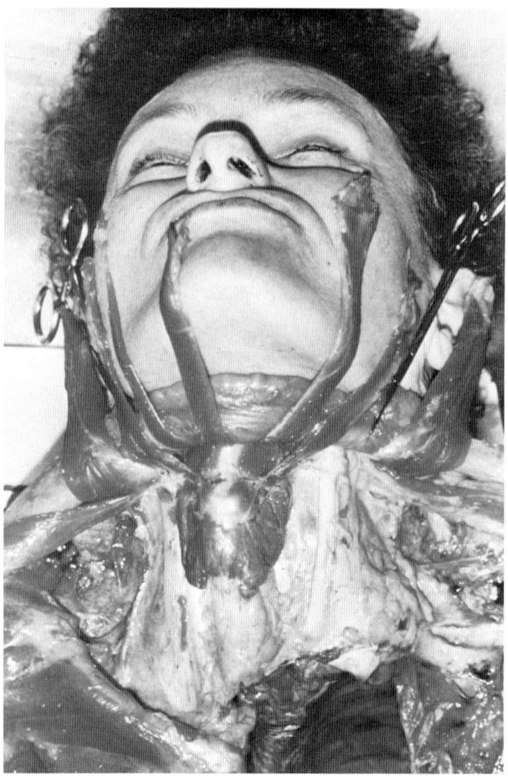

Figure 2.36 An *in situ* dissection of the neck muscles is necessary in cases of suspected strangulation.

to dissect along the fascial planes. The thyroid gland is next removed *in toto*. Now the entire trachea and esophagus are reflected upwards and the precervical fascia is examined and photographed. The posterior aspect of the esophagus is inspected next. At this point remove the tongue and all the neck structures between the carotid arteries *en bloc*. The cervical spine is now palpated and inspected.

The tongue is serially sectioned to disclose bitemarks or contusions and to inspect the lingual tonsils for petechiae.

The hyoid bone and thyroid cartilage are next dissected free (Fig. 2.37). The thyroid cartilage is carefully cleared of muscle and other soft tissue and inspected for fractures. Pay particular attention to the soft tissues surrounding the thyroid cornua, since they are frequently hemorrhagic in homicidal strangulation. The thyroid cornua should be carefully inspected for fractures. When doc-

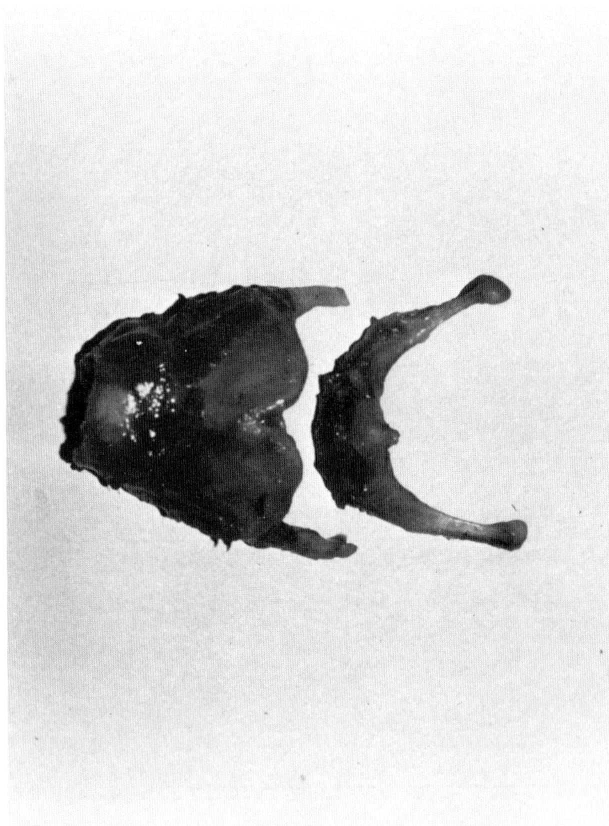

Figure 2.37 The hyoid bone and thyroid cartilage should be cleaned and preserved to document the presence or absence of fractures in cases of suspected strangulation.

umenting fractures, note whether the fracture is beveled medially or laterally and observe the area of the intact periosteum that holds the fractured ends together. Open the larynx posteriorly to inspect the mucosa. Next inspect the soft tissue surrounding the hyoid bone. Remove these tissues and carefully observe the cornua for any fractures. The entire "dissected neck" should be preserved in formalin as evidence to be made available to any future consulting pathologist. This specimen, along with the autopsy protocol and photographs, should be ample material for adequate review if a question arises in the future.

Any hemorrhagic area encountered during the dissection should be sampled microscopically.

FATAL SEXUAL ASSAULT

The sexual assault that may have occurred in a homicide victim may, by itself, result in no physical injuries whatsoever. The pathologist must therefore be suspicious when the scene of death or general profile of the victim suggests that a sexual assault may have occurred. Proper specimens should then be taken, even if the police believe that the motive for a murder is robbery and that no sexual assault took place. The following case is illustrative:

An elderly lady stabbed and strangled was found dead on the floor of the bedroom (Fig. 2.38) of her apartment. She was clad in a sweater, housedress, bra, and panties. The panties were perfectly in place. The assailant, a disgruntled repairman, was later apprehended and confessed not only to the murder but also to raping the victim. He indicated that he had vaginal intercourse with her by simply pushing her panties aside, thereby exposing her introitus without removing the undergarment. Subsequently, a vaginal examination of the deceased revealed a contusion and abrasion of the vagina near the introitus.

In this case, specimen collection (of hair, blood, vaginal washings, etc.) may well have been ignored, since the scene did not obviously suggest a rape had occurred, her clothing was on and intact, and no obvious perineal trauma was evident.

The pathologist should therefore be familiar with the general profile of the rape/murder. The female victim often dies from mechanical asphyxiation. Weapons used are generally those readily available at the scene and often reflect the emotionality and impulsiveness of the act. Older women (averaging 51 years of age) are more often found dead at home, whereas younger women (averaging 31 years of age) are more frequently found in isolated outdoor areas. Also encountered are torn clothing, varying degrees of disrobing, ligature binding, bitemarks, and acute ethanol intoxication.

Whenever a female is found murdered by stabbing, strangulation, bludgeoning, or other manual means, a "rape workup" is necessary. Also do this for

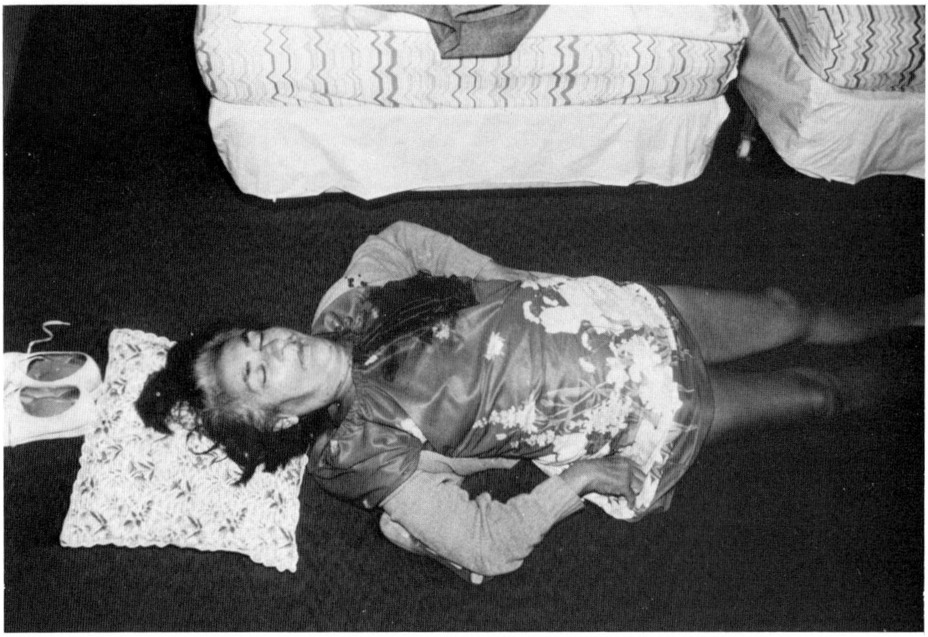

Figure 2.38 Mere suspicion of the possibility of sexual assault should initiate appropriate testing and evidence collection. This murder victim was sexually assaulted. The neatness of the scene and the undisturbed clothing at first misled investigators. The perpetrator merely pushed the underclothing aside to gain vaginal penetration.

males who die in all-male institutions (jails, schools, etc.) and when "overkill" is evident because of numerous forcible injuries. Valuable evidence may otherwise be lost.

Children as well may fall victim to fatal sexual assault. This should be considered not only in obvious cases but also in any unwitnessed death where the child is found in a remote area. Even under apparently innocent death circumstances, at least the external aspects of the genitalia and anus should be carefully inspected for signs of trauma. Since questions of forcible rape are often considered by parents even in unlikely circumstances, this simple examination may allay their fears if nothing else.

In the homicide victim suspected of being sexually assaulted, three kinds of evidence must be considered: (1) evidence for manual or ligature strangulation; (2) bitemarks, if present; and (3) serological and other evidence of sexual assault. Strangulation and bitemarks are dealt with on pages 92 through 98. Procedures for the collection of serologic, microscopic, and other evidence of sexual assault are outlined in the remainder of this chapter.

It is important to remember that clothing may also contain serologic evidence and must be carefully inspected and dried as soon as possible. All serologic specimens must be collected before the body is washed. If photographs are obtained prior to specimen collection, be sure the photograph labels do not contact those areas from which serologic specimens are to be collected (e.g., vaginal introitus, mouth, anus). Generally, photographs with rulers and accession numbers can be taken after the collection of serologic materials. Photographs of the mouth, the genitals, and the anal region should be taken even if no signs of trauma are present. ''Pertinent negatives'' are as appropriate as documentation of real trauma.

The materials needed for specimen collection are contained in a prepackaged ''rape kit'' (Fig. 2.39). The specimens to be collected and the procedures for obtaining them are as follows:

Hands: The fingernails should be scraped for evidence of foreign blood or hairs. Collection is best done at the scene, or the hands may be covered with paper bags (not plastic) for subsequent sampling in the morgue.

Hair: 1. Comb the pubic area for evidence of foreign hairs. Submit the combings and the entire comb in a sealed labeled paper bag.

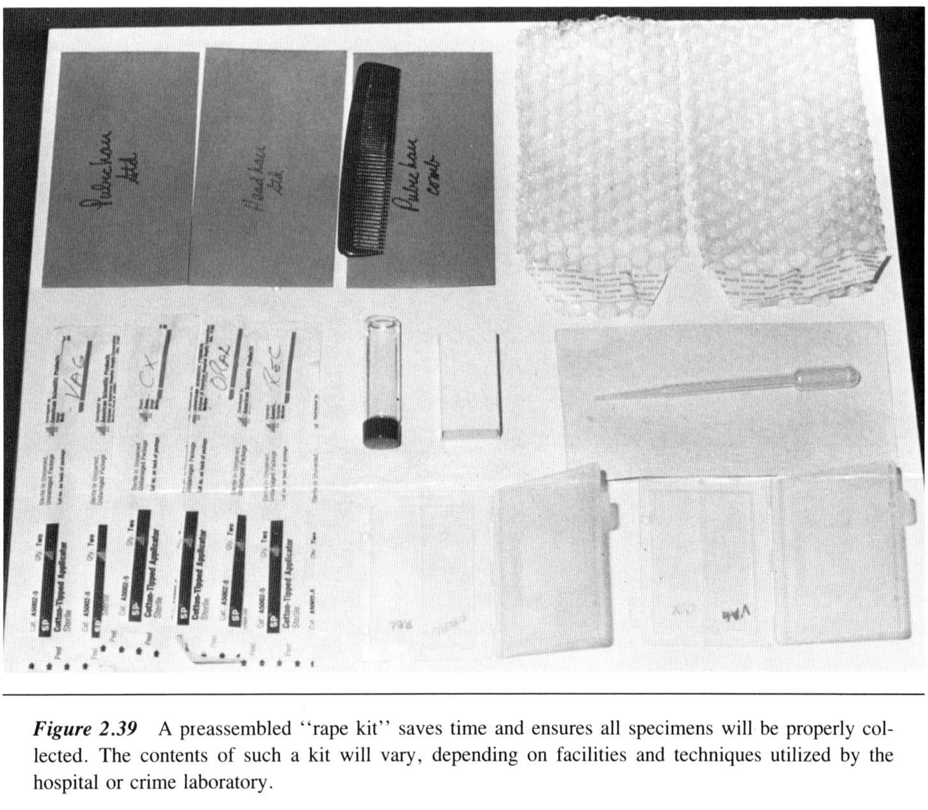

Figure 2.39 A preassembled ''rape kit'' saves time and ensures all specimens will be properly collected. The contents of such a kit will vary, depending on facilities and techniques utilized by the hospital or crime laboratory.

2. Obtain 20–25 pubic hairs by pulling them from different parts of the vulva and place them in an appropriately labeled envelope. Never cut the hairs, since examination of the roots may be of importance.
3. Obtain 20–25 head hairs by pulling them from different parts of the head and place them in an appropriately labeled envelope.

Oral Specimens:

1. A saliva control must be obtained by swabbing the buccal mucosa with a cotton swab and then retaining the swab in its original container. We have found that commercially available sterile cotton swabs may be utilized and the specimen returned to its original container. The paper container permits aeration of the specimen and thereby prevents overgrowth of bacteria. The specimen container should only be opened minimally and then sealed with an adhesive label. Sterile rubber gloves should be used while taking the sample to avoid contamination by your sweat, etc.
2. Utilizing a sterile cotton-tipped swab from an appropriately labeled container, sample the surface of the tongue and the anterior portion of the buccal mucosa between the lips and gingiva. After obtaining the specimen, an appropriately labeled glass slide is smeared, permitted to dry, and subsequently examined for spermatozoa. The swabs are then placed back into the original, appropriately labeled container and subsequently tested for acid phosphatase.

Anal Specimens: The anus, anal canal, and distal portion of the rectum are sampled for spermatozoa and acid phosphastase by utilizing swabs from the appropriately labeled container. The swabs are then smeared on a labeled glass slide and permitted to dry. The swabs are placed back into the original appropriately labeled container.

Vaginal and Cervical Specimens:

1. An autopsy block may be placed under the buttocks to facilitate the examination. Use a clean, preferably sterile speculum. Utilizing swabs from the appropriately labeled containers, sample the vagina and cervix. Smears must be made on appropriately labeled glass slides and permitted to dry. The swabs are placed back into the original, appropriately labeled container.
2. If at least 2 ml of vaginal fluid is present, this should be aspirated with a plastic pipette and placed in an empty screw-capped test tube. (Note: screw-capped tubes are often better than stoppered tubes, since gases sometimes

form in the containers and the pressure may dislodge the stopper.)

3. If less than 2 ml of fluid is within the vagina, obtain vaginal washings. Five milliliters of sterile saline is deposited in the vagina and the fluid is flushed over as much surface area as possible with a plastic pipette. The fluid should be mixed several times by repeated aspiration and then placed in a screw-capped tube.
   Note: Cervical and vaginal smears are always collected before the vaginal aspirate or washings.

Other Body Areas: Other body areas that are suspicious for deposits of seminal fluid should have smears and swabs prepared. A Wood's light may be utilized (ultraviolet light) to detect deposits of seminal fluid. Specifically search the lower abdomen, pubic area, and anterior and medial portions of the thighs.

Blood: One screw-capped tube of blood without any preservative is collected. The specimens should be stored at 4 degrees centigrade if delivery to the crime laboratory is delayed. The specimens are to be saved in a paper bag, which is properly closed with an attached property receipt. Never use plastic bags, since they are airtight, retain moisture, and promote bacterial and fungal growth. A blood sample should be stored separately from the other specimens to avoid contamination.

The saliva control is for detection of the secretor status of the victim, and the blood sample is submitted for grouping and enzyme typing. The vaginal aspirate (or washings) should be examined for the presence of motile sperm. The aspirate and swabs are tested for acid phosphatase, and the smears are stained and screened for the presence of spermatozoa.

The order of specimen collection is extremely important: while the body is supine, samples of scalp and pubic hair are obtained, and oral samples (smears, saliva) may be collected as well as smears from the anterior-medial thighs and lower abdomen. Use of ultraviolet light (Wood's lamp) is useful in identification of seminal fluid on the skin of the thighs and elsewhere. The body should then be turned over (prone) for examination and specimens collected from the anal region. The anal region is examined before the vulva and vagina, since vaginal washings may contaminate the anal and perineal area.

After all specimens have been collected, the skin may be cleaned for photography and subsequent autopsy. A neck dissection should be performed in each and every case of suspected sexual assault for evidence of possible strangulation, even in the presence of an obvious cause of death (e.g., multiple stab wounds). During the examination of the abdominal cavity and pelvis, look for evidence of traumatic perforation of the vagina or anus. The vulva, vagina,

Table 1 Rape Kit Contents

Item	Purpose
3 small envelopes	Scalp and pubic hair standards
1 comb[1]	Pubic hair combings
5 swabs (2 each in container)[2]	Saliva control; oral, anal, cervical and vaginal swabs
4 glass slides with cardboard or plastic slide holders	Oral, anal, cervical and vaginal smears
Pipette	Vaginal washings
1 screw-capped bottle with 5 ml sterile saline[3]	Vaginal washings
1 vaginal speculum	Vaginal examination
1 10-ml preservative-free blood collection tube[4]	Blood standard for serologic testing and typing
Labels	Affix to specimens
2 paper bags	Transport and storage of kit contents

[1]Place comb directly in envelope labeled Pubic Combings.
[2]Swabs stored in their original paper containers (instead of plastic) permit adequate drying and tend to inhibit bacterial contamination.
[3]The screw-capped bottle helps prevent leakage.
[4]Submit blood standard separately to avoid contamination, or use screw-capped container.

internal genitalia, anus, and distal rectum should be inspected after *en bloc* removal (Fig. 2.40). If any injury is detected, consider if it is likely to have resulted from forcible intercourse (particularly in elderly women) or from instrumentation (e.g., insertion of a stick into the vagina). Examine the mucosa of the anus and rectum for any material that may resemble seminal fluid. These areas should be sampled with swabs for the detection of acid phosphatase and spermatozoa.

Male homicide victims suspected of being sexually assaulted, or who may have died during or after a homosexual act, should have the same specimens collected except, of course, for the genitalia. The penis should be swabbed for the detection of saliva (salivary amylase and secretor protein). The detection of sperm or acid phosphatase on the male genitalia is meaningless, since seminal emission is common in the early postmortem state (an effect of rigor mortis).

Although the chances of finding spermatozoa or acid phosphatase are greatly diminished in mildly or moderately decomposed bodies, specimens should still be collected, since a positive result is of great importance.

One cautionary note is in order. The absence of sperm or acid phosphatase does not indicate aspermia or that a sexual assault did not occur. Reportedly, about 30% of rapists do not ejaculate at the time of the assault.

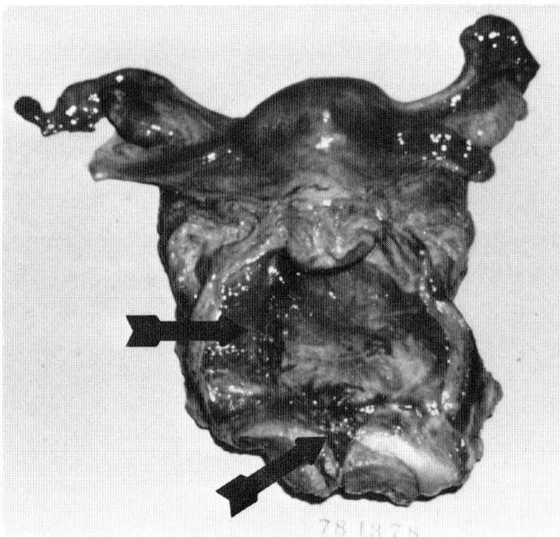

Figure 2.40 *En bloc* removal of the internal genitalia of female victims of sexual assault permits adequate inspection as well as photographic and histologic documentation. Note sutured laceration along the right side of the vaginal wall and the posterior wall anteriorly (arrows).

NONFATAL SEXUAL ASSAULT

The victim of a nonfatal sexual assault has been sexually, emotionally, and physically traumatized. Remember that these victims may well be going through a grief reaction with various stages of denial (including denial of facts or consequences) and anger. They need empathy and support from both the nurse and the examining physician. Judgmental comments are totally inappropriate, even if, in your opinion, "She asked for it." A rapport is essential to a successful evaluation and treatment.

Response time to the emergency room should be without delay, since sperm, acid phosphatase, and serologic markers (blood groups, secretor substances, etc.) disappear with time.

A very brief history of the assault and the assailant is taken for the sole purpose of orienting you as to what tests, procedures, and treatment may be necessary. A detailed account of the events will be taken by the appropriate police investigator.

The date of the last menstrual period should be obtained. If the victim is at mid-cycle, diethylstilbestrol (DES) and trimethobenzamide (Tigan®) are administered. Also obtain the date of the last consensual intercourse. This aids in the interpretation of test results (sperm and acid phosphatase). Furthermore, if the victim had sexual intercourse with her husband or boyfriend during that time, and may be in the early stages of pregnancy, DES is contraindicated because of its teratogenic effects. Subsequent abortion must then be considered. Also obtain any history of venereal disease or hepatitis, which may help interpret laboratory results or guide treatment, prophylactic or otherwise.

The time and date of the assault are important. If the assault occurred within 48 hours prior to the examination, then appropriate specimens for evidence are taken (Fig. 2.41). If the assault took place more than 48 hours earlier, specimens are not taken, but prophylactic treatment in the form of procaine penicillin or spectinomycin or rocephin is given. Cultures for gonorrhea and blood drawn for a serologic test for syphilis are sent to the public health laboratory.

Questions pertaining to the assailant are important to the investigation: whether he is known or unknown to the victim, whether there were threats, restraints, or weapons used. Often a rapist is a repeat offender with a similar mode of operation each time, which aids in his apprehension. These questions, however, should not be overly detailed, since you are not a police detective. The information is for the sole purpose of directing your examination.

If the patient has physical injuries, these are recorded on body diagrams, noting the type of injury, the dimensions, etc. Pay particular attention to the sound of the voice (viz., hoarseness), neck injuries, and bulbar petechiae, since sexual assault victims are often strangled. If warranted, X-rays and/or a surgical consult should be obtained.

The patient's genitalia are then examined after placing her in the lithotomy position. If the patient has not washed, bathed, or douched, the pubic hair is combed using a fresh, unused comb. The comb and combings are placed in an envelope that is appropriately labeled and sealed. If there is visible foreign material on her body (grass, dirt, weeds, etc.) from the scene of the assault, this should also be impounded as corroborative evidence.

The vaginal area is swabbed. Use two cotton-tipped swabs. Make a vaginal smear and replace the swabs into the labeled paper container. Next swab the cervical area in a similar fashion. The vagina and cervical area are then washed using 2 ml of sterile saline. Using a plastic pipette, the fluid is taken up and squirted over the vaginal vault and then aspirated and placed into an appropriately labeled container. A culture for gonorrhea is taken by placing a sterile cotton-tipped swab within the cervical canal and gently pressing against the sides of the cervix. It is then plated on a chocolate agar plate. A pap smear is then taken and screened for sperm as well as for herpetic changes and other cytologic abnormalities.

If there has been attempted anal sex, this orifice is next examined for injury using a disposable plastic anoscope. Swabs and smears are obtained along with a culture for gonococcus.

If there has been oral sex, swabs and smears are taken of the area anterior and posterior to the front teeth, the gums, under the tongue, and the area of the hard palate. A gonococcal culture is taken from the hypopharyngeal and tonsillar area.

The patient then chews on a small piece of cotton, making it wet with saliva, and the specimen is placed in a small cardboard box without handling it at any

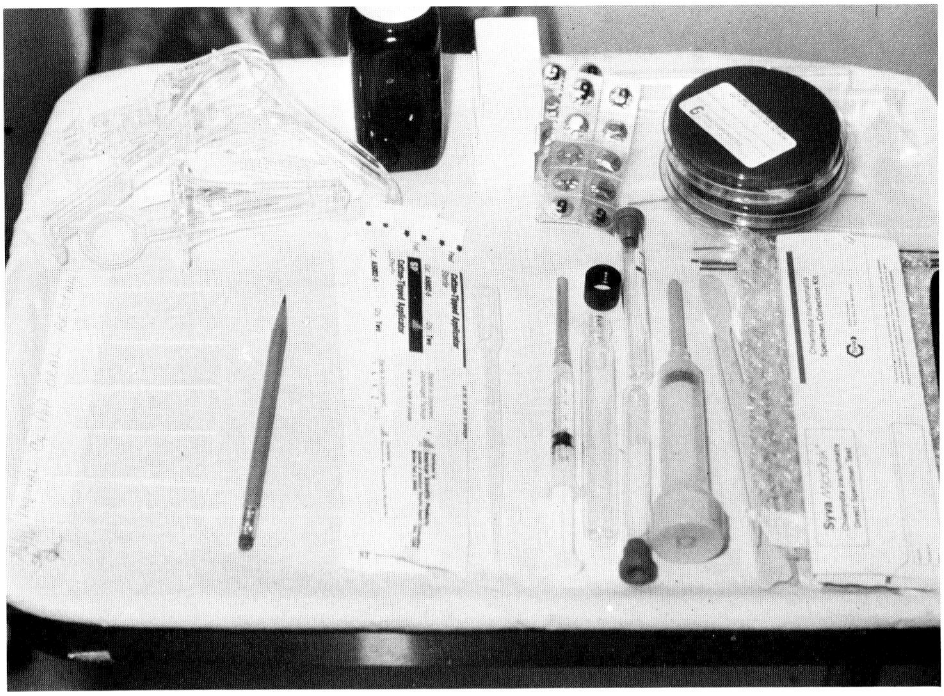

Figure 2.41 Items needed for the examination of a victim of nonfatal sexual assault.

Disposable plastic speculum or a metal speculum
2 vaginal swabs (1 pkt)
2 cervical swabs (1 pkt)
1 vaginal slide
1 cervical slide
2 rectal swabs
2 oral swabs
1 rectal slide
1 oral slide
Vaginal aspirate—2 cc sterile saline in bottle with pipette
Saliva control—piece of sterile cloth in small box
Blood tube for typing
Comb for pubic hair combings
Envelope for collecting possible foreign material on victim
Brown paper bag to hold above evidence

Cultures

Chocolate agar plates (gonococcus)
Chlamydia trachomatis kit when available
Swabs for procurement of above specimens
Pap smear—bottle with fixative and spatula to take specimen—glass slide

time. The box is labeled as saliva control and used to evaluate the victim's blood group and secretor status, if applicable.

The vaginal aspirate is next examined microscopically for the presence of sperm, noting any motility if sperm are observed. If sperm are not present, then a visual test for acid phosphatase is done.

Blood samples are submitted for a VDRL and for serologic testing of blood groups. All specimen labels are initialed by the physician who took them and

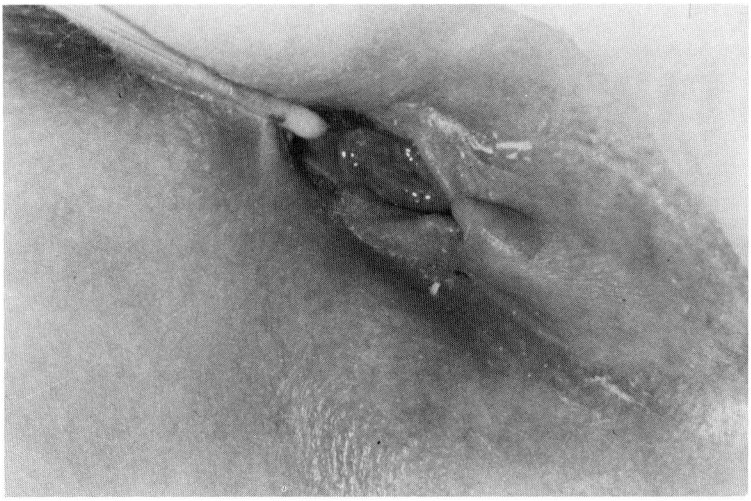

Figure 2.42 Intact hymenal ring, with no trauma. Smooth margins.

glass slides are signed with pencil. All specimens are placed in a paper bag, sealed with evidence tape, and handed over to the detective. If a police officer is not at the examining center, then the paper bag is placed in a specially designated, secured refrigerator.

In females presumed to have been virginal prior to the assault, specific attention must be directed to the hymenal ring. Note its overall configuration, whether it is torn, or has healed tears (Figs. 2.42 and 2.43).

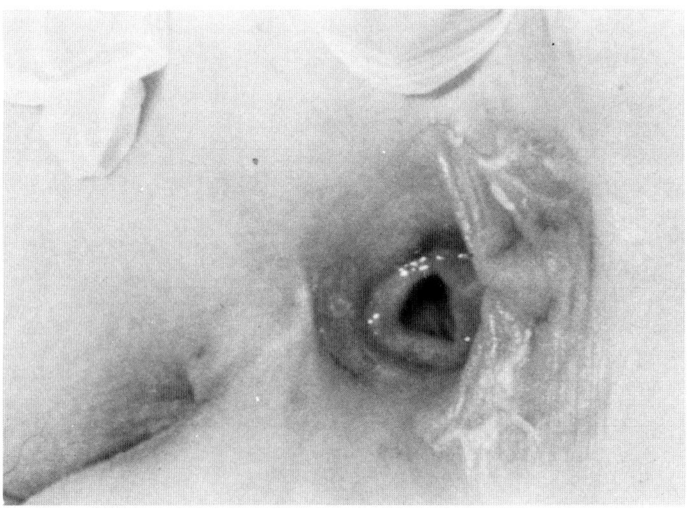

Figure 2.43 Irregular, notched (at 11, 2, and 6 o'clock positions) hymenal ring with marked edema. Irregularity is due to healed old tears, probably due to digital penetration.

RAPE TREATMENT CENTER

JACKSON MEMORIAL HOSPITAL UNIVERSITY OF MIAMI SCHOOL OF MEDICINE

PATIENTS ADDRESS ______

PLACE OF EXAM ______ DATE: ______

TIME: ______

PERSONAL HISTORY

PARA ___ ___ ___ ___ GR. ______

LMP: DATE ______ NORMAL ABNORMAL

LAST COITUS: DATE ______ TIME: ______

CONTRACEPTION: YES NO TYPE: ______

DOUCHE BATH DEFECATE VOID DRINK SINCE ASSAULT

VENERAL DISEASE: YES NO TYPE ______ RX ______

HEPATITIS: YES NO WHEN ______ RX ______

HISTORY OF ASSAULT

DATE: ______ TIME: ______

LOCATION: ______

NO. OF ASSAILANTS ______ RACE: B W L O UNK

ATTACKER: KNOWN ______ UNK ______ RELATIVE ______

THREATS: YES NO TYPE ______

RESTRAINTS: YES NO TYPE ______

WEAPON: YES NO TYPE ______

RESIST YES NO

	ORAL	ANAL	VAGINAL	DIGITAL	FOR. BODY
TYPE OF SEX:	___	___	___	___	___
PENETRATION:	___	___	___	___	___
EJACULATION:	___	___	___	___	___

BIRTHDATE ______ RACE ______ M S W D SEP

POLICE DEPT. ______ CASE # ______

OFFICER ______

GENERAL EXAM: (bruises, trauma, lacerations, marks)
NO HISTORY

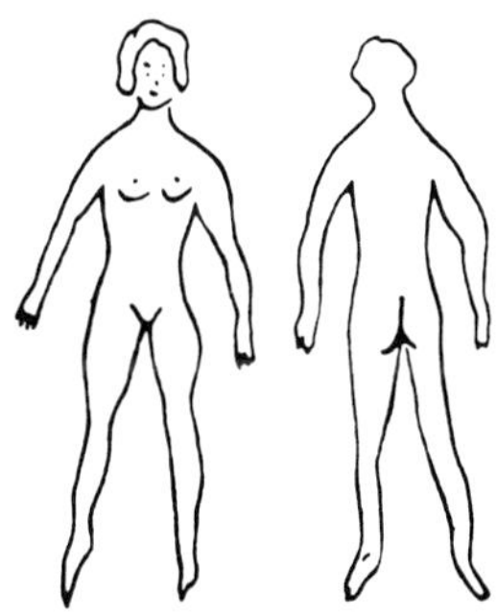

PELVIC EXAM: (include signs of trauma, bleeding, foreign bodies)

VULVA ______

HYMEN ______

VAGINA ______

CERVIX ______

FUNDUS ______

ADNEXAE ______

RECTAL ______

COMMENTS: ______

______

______

______

______

______

PAGE 1 **SEXUAL BATTERY FORM**

RAPE TREATMENT CENTER

MIAMI, FLORIDA

JACKSON MEMORIAL HOSPITAL UNIVERSITY OF MIAMI SCHOOL OF MEDICINE

PHYSICIAN ______ NURSE ______ COUNSELOR ______

HEIGHT ______ WEIGHT ______

TESTS

GC CULTURE: ORAL ANAL CERVICAL OTHER ______

VDRL: YES NO (5cc venous blood - red top)

PAP TEST: YES NO

TREATMENT

V.D. PROPHYLAXIS: YES NO TYPE ______

PREGNANCY PROPHYLAXIS: YES NO TYPE ______

TETANUS: YES NO OTHER MEDS: ______

EVIDENTIAL SPECIMENS, TESTING AND RECEIPT

RESULTS OF PRELIMINARY TESTS: A.P.: NEGATIVE WEAK MODERATE STRONG

SPERM (PER H.P.F.): NONE 1-5 6-10 10+ MOTILE NON-MOTILE

SPECIMENS OBTAINED:	GIVEN TO POLICE	OTHER TREATMENT
10 cc VENOUS BLOOD (red top) ______	______	X-RAY ______
FINGER NAIL SCRAPINGS ______	______	SURGICAL CONSULT ______
PUBIC HAIR COMBINGS ______	______	PSYCH. CONSULT ______
VAGINAL SMEAR ______	______	OTHER: (Explain) ______
VAGINAL SWAB ______	______	
CERVICAL SMEAR ______	______	______
CERVICAL SWAB ______	______	
VAGINAL ASPIRATE ______	______	______
RECTAL SMEAR ______	______	______
RECTAL SWAB ______	______	
ORAL SMEAR ______	______	______
ORAL SWAB ______	______	
SALIVA SPECIMEN ______	______	GIVEN TO POLICE

CLOTHING (number)______ TYPE ______ CONDITION ______

FOREIGN BODIES (number)______ TYPE ______ LOCATION ______

OTHER SPECIMENS______

PHOTOGRAPHS: YES NO TAKEN BY______

TOTAL NUMBER SPECIMENS **TOTAL TO POLICE**

RECEIPT OF EVIDENCE: THE ABOVE EVIDENCE HAS BEEN RECEIVED BY ME ON (DATE) ______ AT (TIME)______ (OFFICER'S SIGNATURE)______

PHYSICIAN'S SIGNATURE:______

WITNESS SIGNATURE______

PAGE 2 | **SEXUAL BATTERY FORM**

Finally, a notation is made about the patient's overall demeanour during the examination (crying, upset, angry, etc.). You may need to refer to this during subsequent criminal proceedings. All records and laboratory results are kept in the strictest confidence and made available only to the prosecuting attorney and investigating police agency.

A followup appointment at 6 weeks is made for the patient, at which time the cultures and a VDRL are redrawn and a pelvic examination is done. Counselling appointments are also made for the victim.

BITEMARK EVIDENCE

The obvious defense for a fingerprint left at a crime scene is for the suspect to state he was there a day or a week before the incident. Today, not only may a bitemark left on a homicide victim be linked to a specific person (assailant), but the odontologist can testify that it was inflicted "at or about the time of death" (because of preserved indentations and the lack of swelling). The suspect must now answer a question such as, "What were your teeth doing on her buttocks at or about the time of death?" Even if the wounds are only "consistent with" or "do not exclude" the suspect, such evidence is often helpful in court. If the assailant is unknown, other valuable information may also be obtained: estimates of age, race, and sex may sometimes be made, as well as the position of the assailant's mouth. Even the secretor status and blood group of the assailant may be determined. The recognition and proper preservation of bitemark evidence, therefore, cannot be overemphasized.

The following steps are utilized in the collection of bitemark evidence. Although they are idealized and assume the interaction of a forensic odontologist, they can be modified according to one's circumstances. The steps to be taken are:

1. Recognition that the wound is, in fact, a bitemark.
2. Collection of serological evidence (e.g., saliva sample).
3. Photography of the bitemark (the most important step after recognition).
4. Collection of the bitemold for preservation of the evidence.
5. Excision of the bitemark for evidence preservation.
6. "Control" bite collection (if indicated).

Bitemarks can be found at any site on the body and may have many different forms. The most common is the bitering, consisting of the anterior incisors and the adjoining teeth of each dental arch (Fig. 2.44). However, a bite may only be in the configuration of a half-ring (Fig. 2.45), in which only one set of incisors

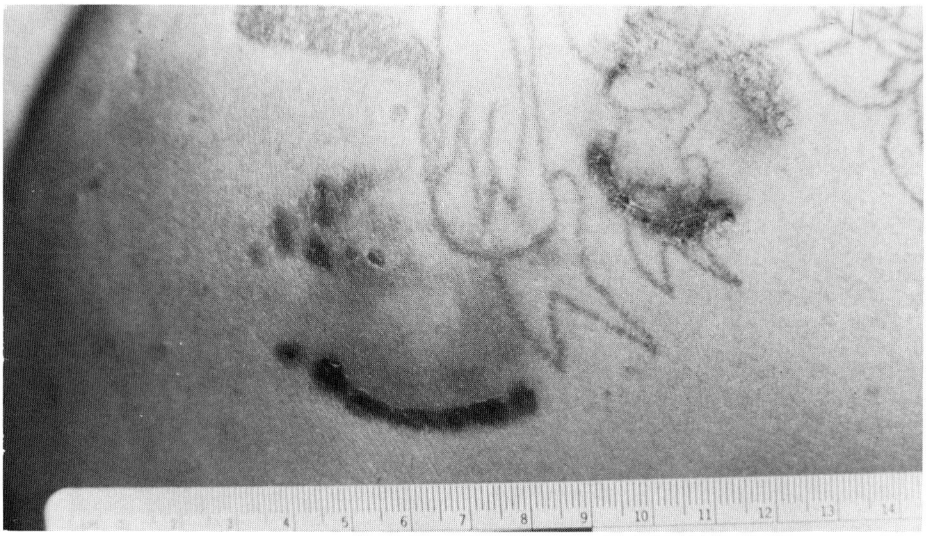

Figure 2.44 The bitering is outlined by abrasions and contusions made by the teeth of the upper and lower dental arches. The two bitemarks (biterings) in this photograph were made by two different assailants.

and adjoining teeth is present, or, in fact, may be a simple, single toothmark (Fig. 2.46). It is important to realize that the bitemark evidence may be left not only on a human body but also on other items at the crime scene. Hungry robbers, after murdering a person, have been known to raid a refrigerator and leave teeth imprints on a slice of bologna.

Once the wound is recognized, it is important to determine whether the bite was from a human or an animal. The canine teeth of animals are quite distinctive and easily recognized.

If the bitemark is identified at the scene of the crime, photography and saliva sample collection may be performed at that time. Closeup photography, however, is usually performed later, at the morgue, under better lighting and working conditions. Handling of the bitemark area must be prohibited if the bitemark workup is to be performed at the morgue. A clean sheet of paper or paper bag (not plastic) should be taped over the bitemark to avoid contamination. The paper should be taped to the area at least 1 inch away from the bitering perimeter. Great effort should be expended to avoid touching the area or contaminating it with blood at the scene. If the victim was bitten through clothing, these items must also be handled so as to avoid contamination.

Once in the morgue, proceed with saliva collection. This is to determine the secretor status of the assailant for comparison with the victim. Also, the detection of salivary amylase helps confirm that the injury or mark was indeed a bitemark. A sterile cotton swab is rubbed on the skin inside the bitering, and a second sterile swab is rubbed on a control site of skin remote from the bitemark. A third swab should be used to obtain a saliva control from the buccal mucosa

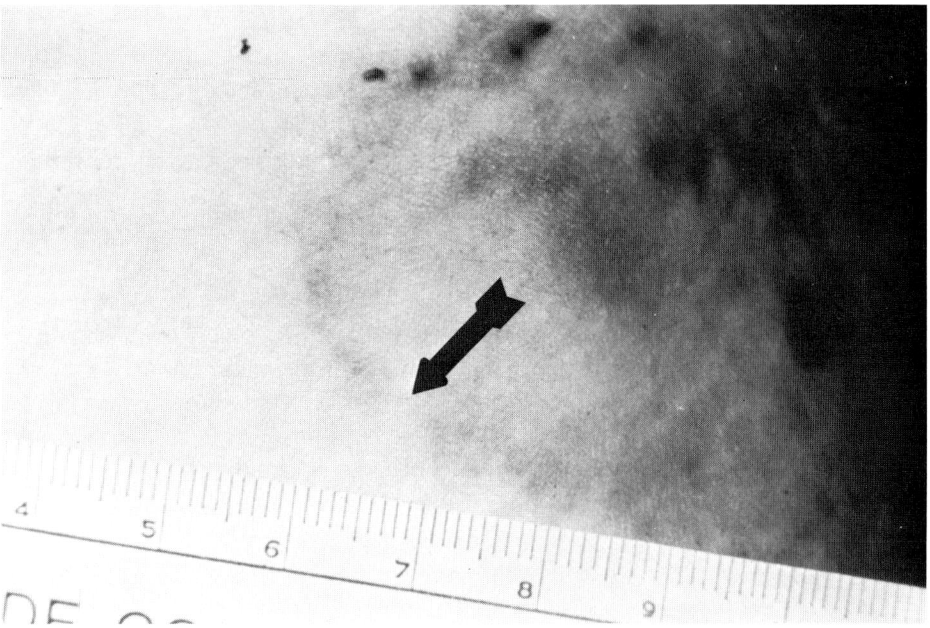

Figure 2.45 A wound made by only one dental arch is called a half-bitering. Note the diastema (arrow) between the imprints of the two front teeth.

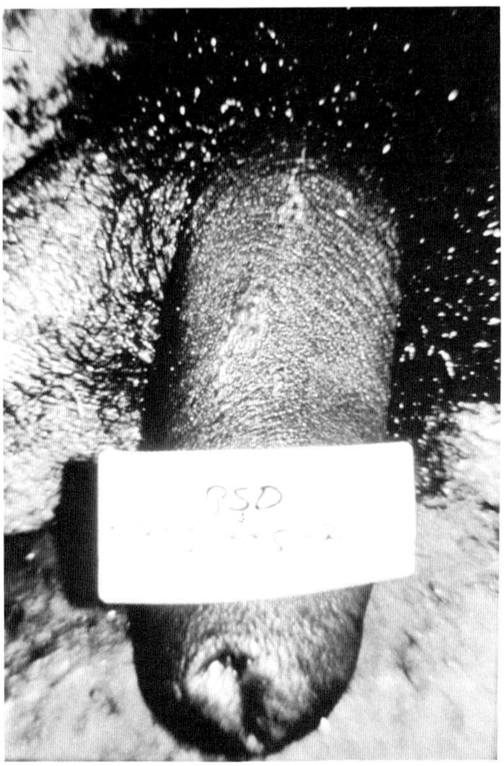

Figure 2.46 A mark from an individual tooth may also have evidentiary value. The toothmark is near the penile base. The more distal abrasion is from sudden withdrawal during forced fellatio. The marks were consistent with sexual assault and not the purported scenario given by the perpetrator. (Photograph courtesy of Richard Souviron, DDS.)

of the victim. If the buccal mucosa is contaminated by blood, a sweat control may be obtained by wetting the sterile swab with sterile saline and swabbing the axillary area. Saliva samples should be obtained before closeup photographs are taken, since all bitemark photographs must be taken with rulers, and therefore there is the possibility of contamination.

The next step in the process is photography. Overview photographs must be taken for proper orientation. Closeup photographs (preferably 1:1) should be obtained with a ruler in both the vertical and the horizontal planes (Fig. 2.47). The ruler should always be in centimeters. A color code is useful in dating the bitemark and may be photographed next to the wound (i.e., a red bitemark indicates a recent wound). Always save a sample of the color code as well as the rulers used in the photographs for quality control when the evidence is reexamined months to years later. For bitemarks, it is worthwhile to take two sets of photographs utilizing two different cameras, since the evidence is so important.

Evidence preservation by fingerprint and bitemold techniques is the next procedure. A technique has been recently developed utilizing fingerprint dusting powder on the bitemark surface. The area is simply dusted with the fingerprint powder, photographed, and then lifted with fingerprint tape. Spectacular models have been obtained with this method (Fig. 2.48).

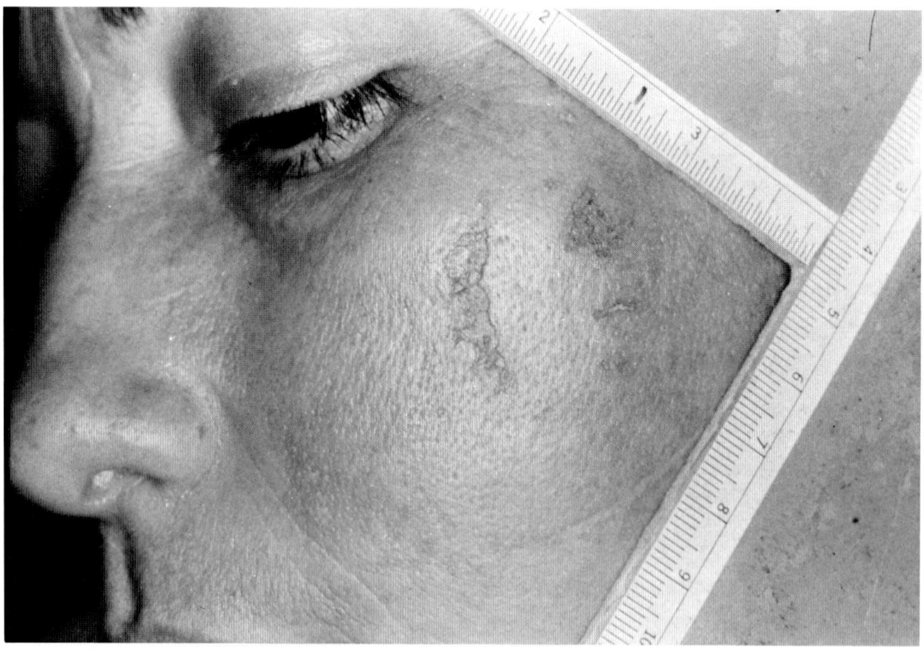

Figure 2.47 Two rulers at right angles are used in photographing the bitemark. Several photographs should be taken with the rulers in various positions. (Photographs courtesy of Richard Souviron, DDS.)

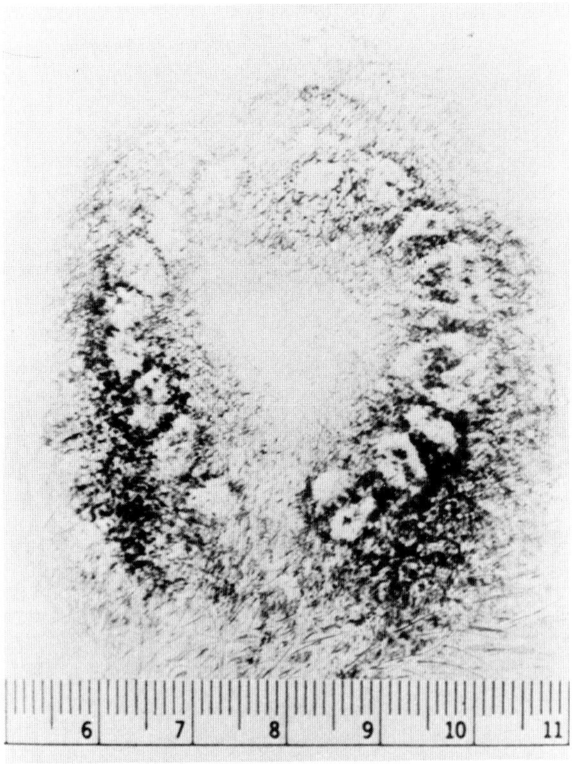

Figure 2.48 A bitemark may be enhanced by dusting with fingerprint powder and "lifted" with clear tape for preservation (reproduced with permission of the American Society of Testing Materials, *J Forensic Sci* 19:326-330, 1984). Reportedly, fingerprint ink has also been successfully utilized for this purpose (personal communication, Dr. Lyvia A. Alvarez, September 1987).

An older, more standard procedure for preserving the bitemark is to make a cast of it. This procedure is described in detail in the Appendix of this chapter. In brief, a light-bodied Permlastic base and catalyst are mixed on a paper mixing pad. This is drawn into a syringe and gently forced into the grooves of the bitemark, upon the surrounding skin, and upon the skin within the bitemark area. The mixture is allowed to harden in place. A dental dye stone is then applied to the surface of the mold for a backing. The mold, with its lasting impression of the bitemark, is then gently lifted from the skin. A reverse mold may then be constructed. Both may later be matched with the assailant's teeth. Equipment including base and catalyst may be purchased from the dental supply house. The mixture is usually put into the syringe by pushing the mouth of the syringe onto the mixture, and then by pushing it into position by the syringe plunger.

After bitemold collection, the bitemark with surrounding skin should be excised and preserved to permit defense experts to examine the bitemark itself.

Simply stated, a square or rectangle of known dimensions is drawn upon the skin surrounding the bitemark. The bitemark is then cut out by excising the outline and stapled onto an identical geometric figure on a thin piece of cardboard. Since the skin is elastic, the specimen must first be stretched out to match the geometric outline and then stapled in place. The bitemark may then be stored in the freezer.

An easier method is to fashion a plastic ring (or other material) around the bitemark and glue it to the skin with cyanoacrylate (Krazy Glue®). Then excise the entire area by cutting the ring (Fig. 2.49).

The last step in the process is to decide whether or not to take an impression of the victim's teeth. This is done if the bitemark is in a place where it could have been self-inflicted. Since obtaining the specimen does require a degree of skill and experience, it is best that a qualified dentist obtain the impression. At the very least, the victim's teeth should be carefully photographed (distant and 1:1 photographs with and without a ruler in place), and an attempt should be made to obtain the dental impressions.

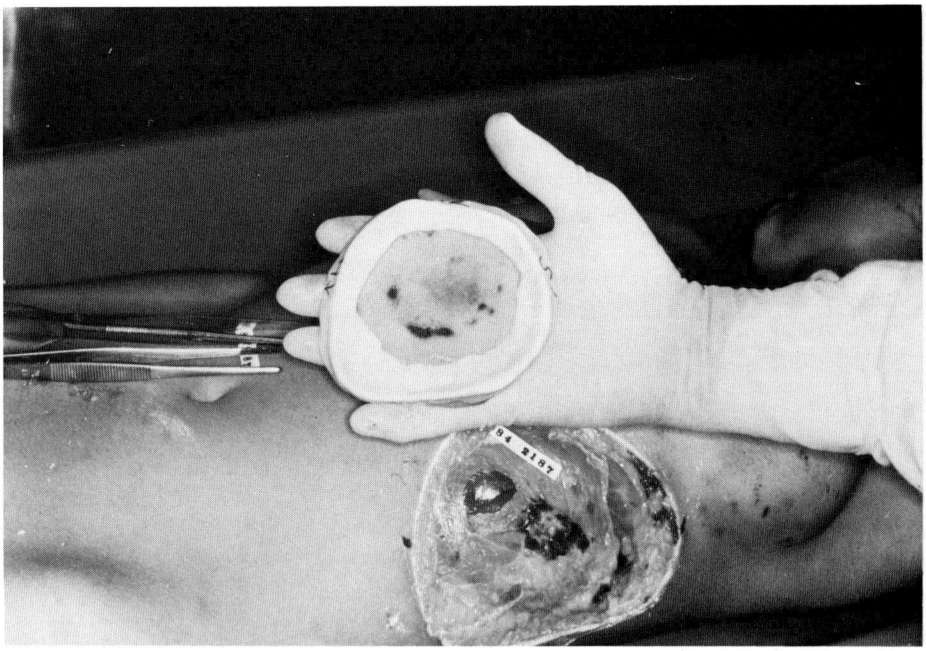

Figure 2.49 The bitemark may be preserved by constructing an acrylic holding ring. Acrylic material (Kerr™ Formatray) is placed around the periphery of the bitemark and allowed to dry upon the skin. The ring is then removed and cyanoacrylate glue is smeared on the surface facing the skin. The ring is replaced around the bitemark and the glue is permitted to dry. The entire bitemark is then extracted by cutting the skin at the outer periphery of the ring. Note: before removing the acrylic ring, be sure to mark the ring with anatomic designations such that it can be placed back on the skin in its original position. (Technique and photograph courtesy of Richard Souviron, DDS.)

If an old bitemark scar is encountered, it should be photographed with as much attention to detail as for a recent bite. The current assailant may well have been the previous one!

The above workup is, of course, ideal, and in real life the practicing pathologist may not have the materials to collect the evidence, nor may there be a dentist available and ready to help. In such circumstances, the saliva collection and numerous photographs should be taken, and then the bitemark should be excised and frozen.

Appendix: Obtaining the Bitemold

The following instructions are reproduced from Souviron R, Mittleman RE, Valor J: Obtaining the bitemark impression (mold) from skin. *FBI Law Enforcement Bulletin* 51:8–11, 1982.

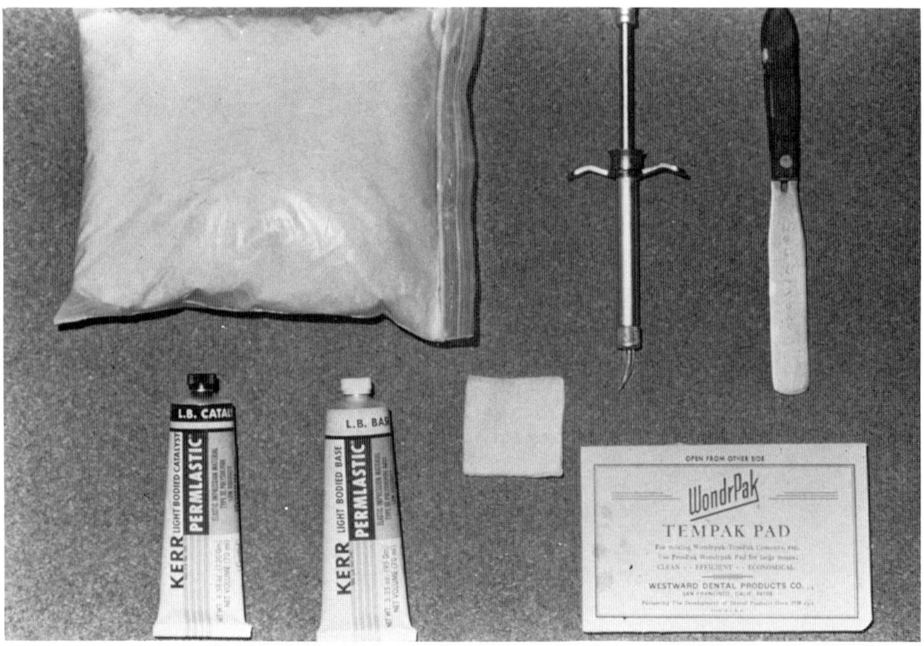

Figure 2.50 *Materials needed*

1) Light-bodied Permlastic base and catalyst
2) Spatula
3) Paper mixing pad
4) Rubber base syringe
5) Gauze (3 × 3-inch square); and
6) Dental dye stone

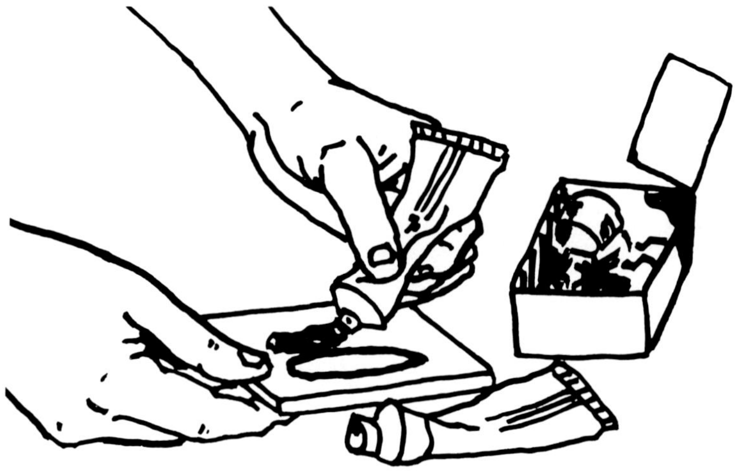

Figure 2.51 Supplies for steps 2–6 can be purchased at any dental supply house.
Method: Squeeze a 2-inch line of both Permlastic base and catalyst onto a sheet of paper mixing pad so that the two lines are parallel to each other, about 1 inch apart.

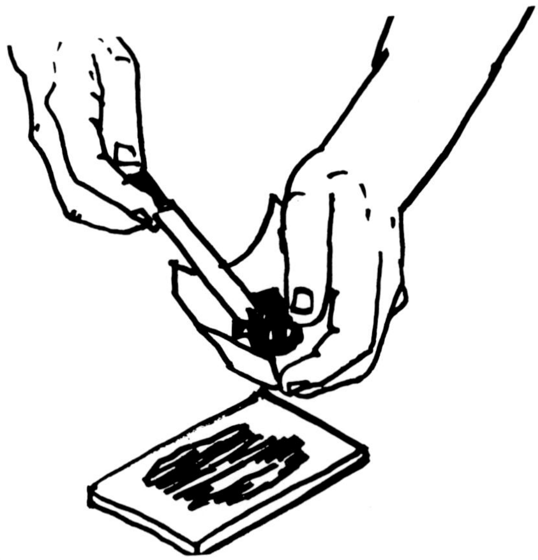

Figure 2.52 Using the spatula, mix the base and catalyst until there is a homogeneous brown color.

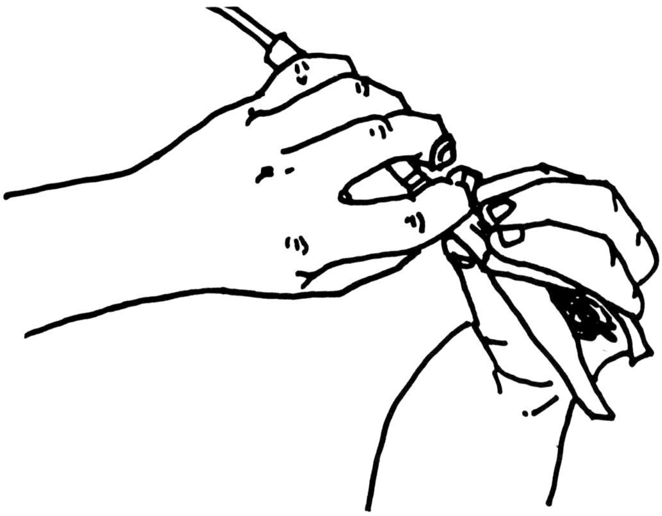

Figure 2.53 Quickly apply to the properly folded sheet from the paper mixing pad and squeeze into the syringe. The syringe package contains instructions for folding, or the syringe barrel may be filled by scraping the barrel across the mixing pad.

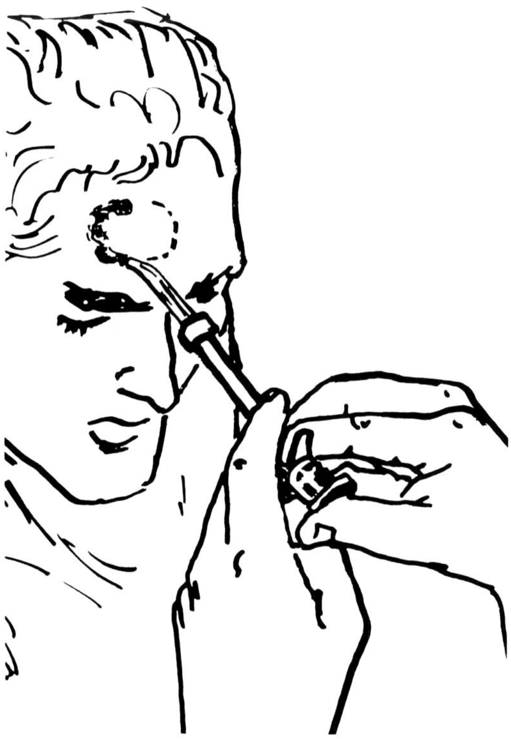

Figure 2.54 Using the rubber base syringe, apply the mixture to the bitemark identations in the skin. It is crucial that air bubbles be avoided. This is accomplished by slowly and methodically beginning at one point within the bitemark ring and continuing the application around the entire ring without stopping. If this is done correctly, the mixture will cover the skin between and around each individual bitemark. It is important to insure that there is a reasonable amount of mixture above the skin level, since the mixture will later be smoothed over the remainder of the skin surface with the spatula.

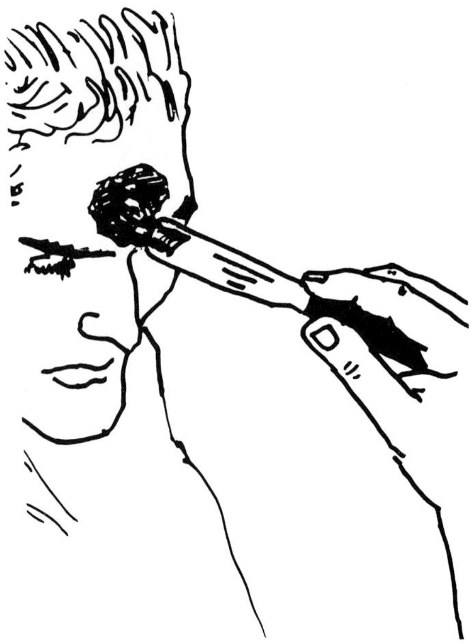

Figure 2.55 Spread mixture over the bitemark area and at least ¼ inch of the adjoining skin from the outer perimeters of the toothmarks. Completely cover the region by spreading the rubber base remaining in the syringe, on the spatula and on the mixing paper.

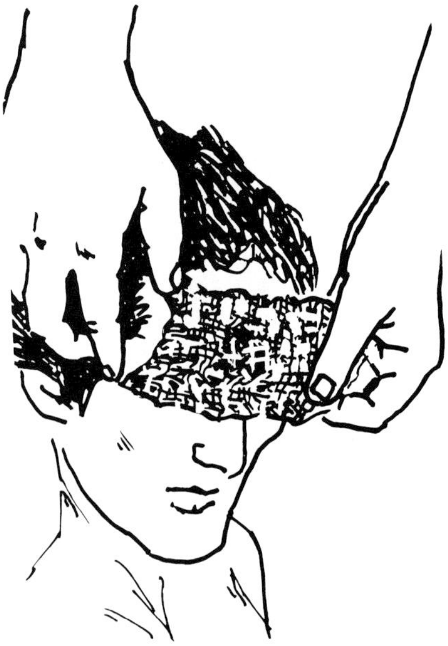

Figure 2.56 Immediately place a single layer of gauze mesh over the area. The gauze should be cut to the appropriate size either before or after placement. It is important that steps 1–5 be completed in a few minutes. Allow the mixture with the gauze to harden for approximately 5 min.

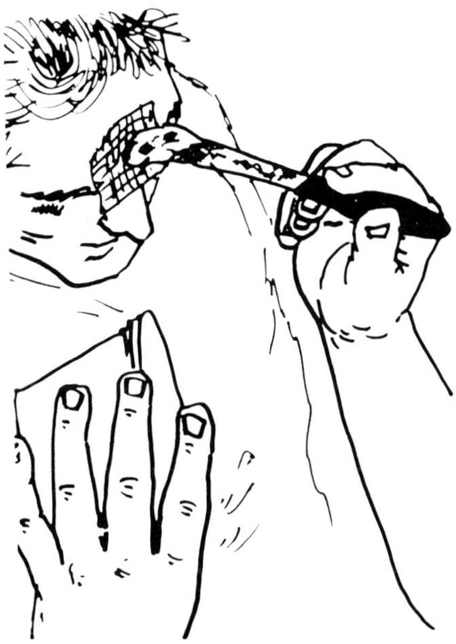

Figure 2.57 Mix dental dye with a small amount of water and place on top of entire surface of gauze. The mixture should be the same consistency as a heavy pancake mix, and the depth of the overlay on the gauze should be about 1 inch. Allow to dry for 15 min.

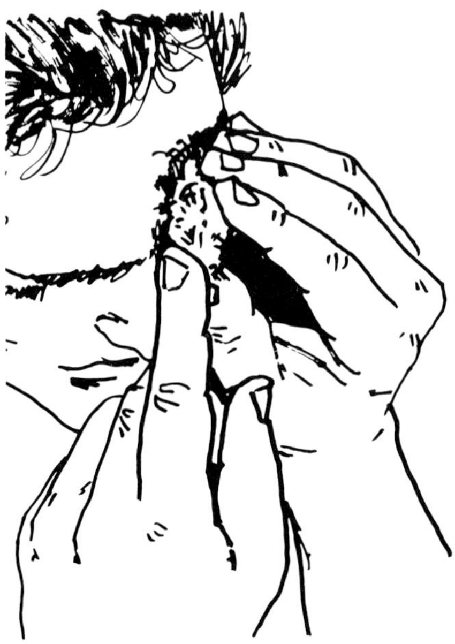

Figure 2.58 The mold should be carefully removed by gently lifting at one end until it is completely removed from the skin surface and should then be stored at room temperature. If there is any evidence of air bubbles, the collecting process should be repeated.

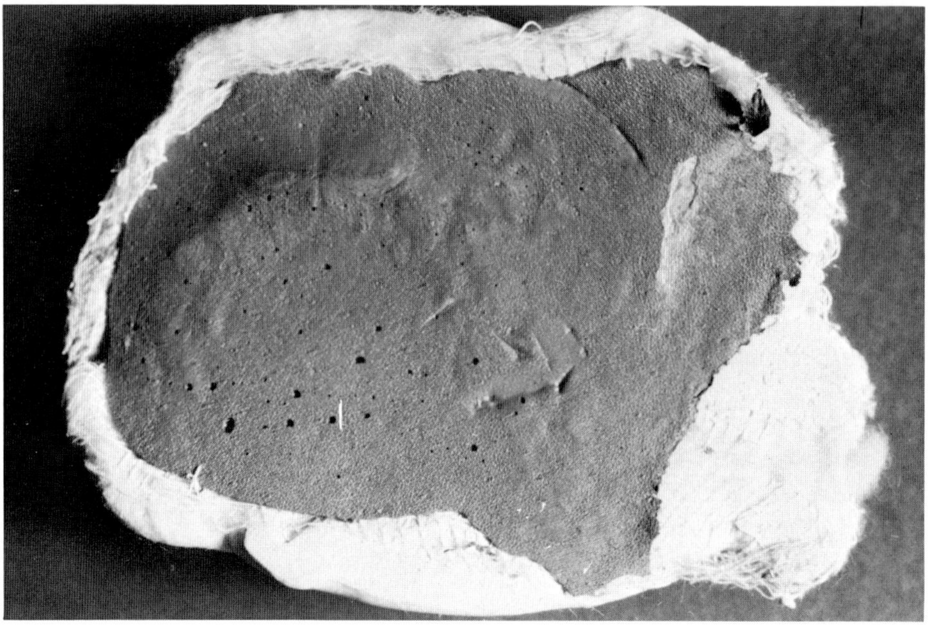

Figure 2.59 The completed bitemold is a permanent record of the impression left on the skin. A reverse mold can be made from this impression for comparison with a suspect's teeth.

FIRE DEATHS

Fire deaths are often the most complicated of forensic cases. The reasons for such challenges are rooted in the fact that both scene and body are invariably disturbed. The scene is usually altered by waves of intruders: firemen, police, medical examiners, and even the curious public. The fire damage itself may well be an ongoing destructive process even after the final flames are extinguished. The deceased can be burned beyond recognition, and investigators may walk past the charred body many times before seeing it. Hence, once the fire is extinguished and human safety assured, the key to all fire deaths is the preservation of the scene for investigation and documentation of any evidence related to the causation of the fire.

The medical examiner should be concerned with the following questions:

1. How did the fire start?
2. Why did it get out of control?
3. Why did the victim not escape?
4. What is the cause and manner of death?
5. Was the victim dead (murdered?) or alive when the fire started?
6. How will the identification of the victim be established?

In general, questions 1 and 2 are answered by fire investigators. The remaining questions are answered by the efforts of many different investigators as well as the pathologist. Constant communication with all those involved in the investigation is crucial.

If the fire was unintentional, the manner of death is usually accidental or natural, depending upon whether or not the fire was the actual cause of death.

Accidental fires are usually attributed to faulty electrical appliances, ignition of combustible materials (pile of gasoline-soaked cleaning rags), ill-placed candles, kitchen and cleaning mishaps, etc. Although scene investigation will usually reveal clues as to the fire's origin, much evidence will have been destroyed by the intense fire and heat. Information about the decedent and the scene prior to the incident may also help establish the cause of the fire. Faulty electrical devices as well as other fire hazards are often known to friends and family members. These informants may also divulge medical or social risk factors of the decedent (e.g., heavy smoker, alcoholic, organic brain syndrome, Parkinson's disease). Certainly the presence of many containers for alcoholic beverages, numerous cigarette butts, as well as certain medications [folic acid, niacin, cerebral vasodilator (Hydergine)] may provide further clues. In most accidental fire deaths, signs of smoke inhalation and fire injury will be evident at the time of autopsy (vide infra). Toxicologic testing for alcohol and other incapacitating drugs is always a major consideration, along with analysis for carbon monoxide and cyanide (generated by the combustion of some plastics).

Natural deaths may result in fire because the victim is no longer alive to control the potential fire hazard (cigarettes, kitchen stove, candles, etc.). Diseases such as atherosclerotic heart disease, cerebrovascular hypertensive complications, and epilepsy are most oten encountered. The autopsy and toxicologic analyses usually do not reveal any evidence whatsoever of smoke inhalation (soot in the airways or carbon monoxide).

Intentional fire deaths may, of course, be the result of arson or suicide. In most suicides, the fire will be centered on or near the victim. In many arson deaths, the victim is at some distance from the origin of the fire and the death is frequently not intended (e.g., derelict residing in an abandoned building that is set on fire to collect the insurance). Nevertheless, the latter is still viewed as homicide by the felony murder rule. Less commonly, accelerant is poured directly onto a victim with homicidal intent. One must always remember that the reason for a fire may be to cremate a murder victim or at least to have the death appear as an accidental fire death to cover up the crime.

In cases of badly charred bodies, attempts at identification should not be based on circumstantial evidence alone if more substantial methods are available. Circumstantial identification may not be honored by courts, insurance companies, or families. Every attempt should therefore be made to identify the victim by comparisons with premortem dental or medical records and X-rays. The teeth must be carefully examined and photographed in all charred bodies. Besides the diagrams, photography with a wide-angle lens is often helpful in delineating the burn pattern.

The body should be photographed in its entirety. Bullet holes are often masked by the fire damage. Hence, all charred bodies should be completely X-rayed for projectiles or fragments that may be discovered radiologically. Also, roentgenograms may well be helpful in establishing the identity of the victim. An autopsy is mandatory in all cases of extensive charring or incineration. At the very least, the autopsy helps to detect or exclude the postmortem incineration of a homicide victim (Figs. 2.60 and 2.61).

The internal examination should be conducted to determine the effects of the fire, and whether or not the person died as a result of the fire. If the organs have a "cherry red" coloration from carbon monoxide, they should be photographed for evidentiary purposes. The upper airways need to be carefully inspected for the presence of soot, which may extend deep into the lungs, and the airways should also be photographed (Figs. 2.62 and 2.63). The autopsy should be conducted to detect any sign of trauma. In charred bodies, where gunshot wounds and stab wounds are not as perceivable externally, careful inspection of the ribs is crucial. In fact, it may well be necessary to remove all tissue from

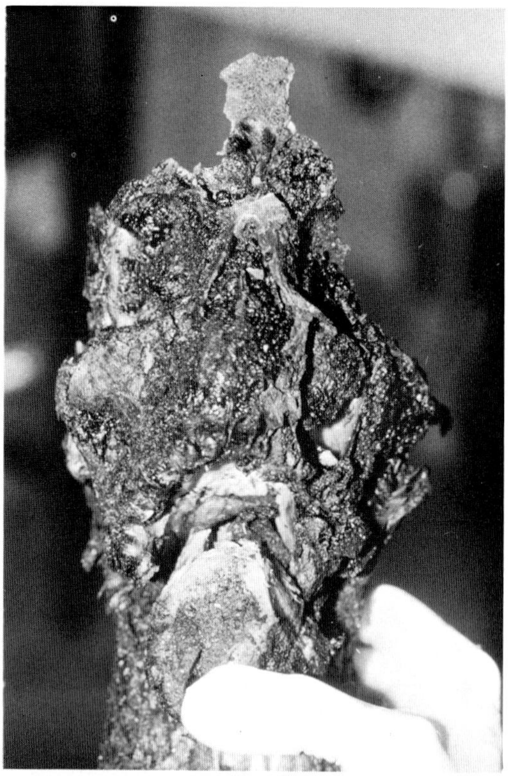

Figure 2.60 This depicts the severely charred remains of a head (frontal view). Despite the damage, an autopsy must be performed. The examination revealed a trail of congealed blood from a gunshot wound.

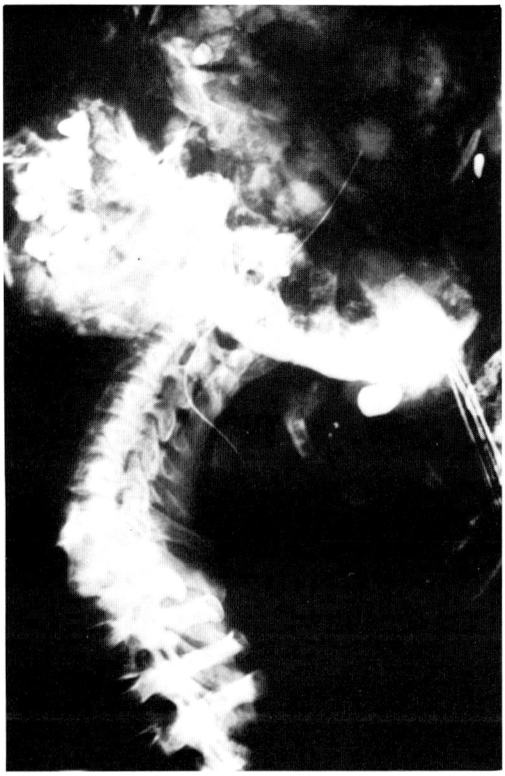

Figure 2.61 Radiologic examination of the charred remains in Fig. 2.60 revealed a bullet in the occipital region. All charred remains must be radiologically examined to exclude homicidal gunshot wounds followed by postmortem incineration.

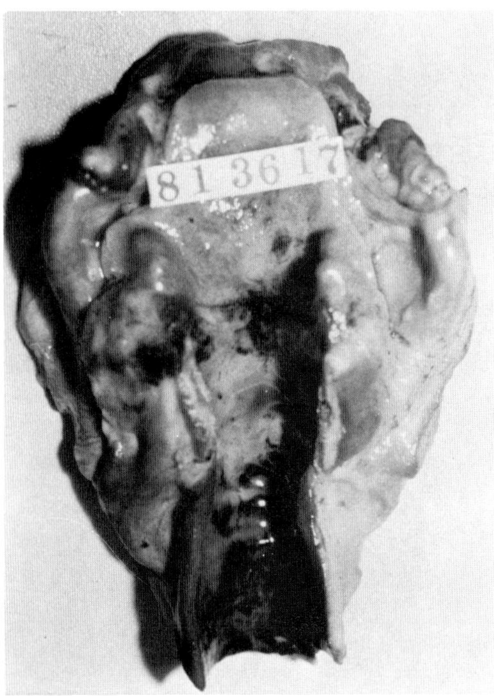

Figure 2.62 Soot in the larynx and trachea should be photographed to help document the person was alive (or probably alive) during a fire.

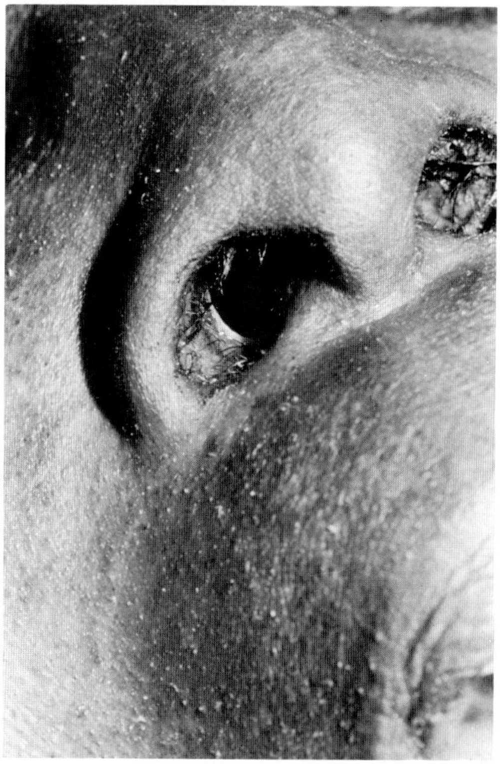

Figure 2.63 Soot in the nostrils may be the only external evidence of smoke inhalation. This person died in a part of a building remote from the actual fire, but nonetheless succumbed to smoke inhalation.

the ribs to ascertain whether or not there are such injuries. Evidence of natural disease should be carefully documented, as it may explain why the decedent could not get out of his situation.

Complete toxicologic testing, especially for carbon monoxide, cyanide, alcohol, and depressant drugs, should be requested. Also, drugs that may result in hallucinations, paranoid reactions, or psychotic behavior may explain the cause of a fire or why the victim did not escape. If blood is not available for carbon monoxide determination, skeletal muscle may be utilized (obtain at least 100 g).

Fire victims may only be covered with soot and, in fact, may have inhaled very little of the carbon monoxide or soot in the atmosphere. This is particularly true if they died from a heart attack or other disease as the fire started. If this is a possibility, specifically examine the nares for the presence of any soot.

Burn victims who die in a hospital at some time after the incident are usually autopsied much as other hospital patients once the photographs are taken and body diagrams are made. First-, second-, and third-degree burns are not appropriate designations for autopsy protocols. It is best simply to describe the injuries rather than to compete with the clinician's assessment. The clinician has the benefit of seeing the burns firsthand rather than days later, as the pathologist often does. Soot deposits may remain in the nares or upper airway (or lungs), depending on the length of survival.

ELECTRICAL DEATHS

All electrical deaths require a detailed analysis of the terminal event and an evaluation of the electrical source. It is also important to be sure that nobody else uses a faulty electrical appliance! Civil litigants and the family will want to know if the equipment was faulty, if there were errors or violations of procedure, and whose fault it was. In all forms of electrocution, anticipate questions concerning the likely or probable position of the victim at the time of the incident (i.e., what was the most likely pathway of the electricity through the body). Specific attention to injury patterns and the clothing is helpful in correlating what happened at the scene of death.

High-Voltage Electrocution

High-voltage electrocutions (in excess of 1,000 volts) usually result when contact is made with a high-power line, and therefore often occur in an industrial or workplace setting. Since these power lines are not insulated, any direct or indirect contact by a grounded person results in electrocution (note: workers in ''cherry pickers'' are insulated but not grounded; hence they can safely work with these lines). Contact is often made by tall, heavy equipment, such as the boom of a crane. The crane is insulated and therefore the operator will not be hurt. But a person on the ground who touches the crane will be electrocuted.

Death from such incidents usually is associated with prominent burns with typical histologic features. Charring is often prominent. Although external examination may not reveal definitive entrance and exit points, the diagrammed and photographed distribution of these injuries allows for future correlation. Clothing and shoes are also helpful for this purpose.

Labeled histologic sections of measured entrance and exit points at least establish that the injury was acute and electrical (i.e., not a preexisting injury). Also specifically photograph any areas that are burned or charred but have nonsinged hair, indicating the heat effect was from an internal and not an external source. Finally, appropriate tests for alcohol and drugs should be ordered.

Lightning

Lightning bolts contain phenomenal amounts of electricity. Observable injuries, however, range from negligible to nearly total annihilation. Usually, varying patterns of electrical burns are evident on both the clothing and body (Fig. 2.64). If the arborization pattern typical for lightning appears on the skin, it should be photographed immediately, since this change is transient. Examine all metal objects and jewelry for melting or other damage (Fig. 2.65). Metals with iron may become magnetized, and this can be demonstrated with a magnetic compass. In those cases where few or no injuries are evident, the possibility of lightning strike must be estimated from the scene and from knowledge of weather conditions. Both the local weather service (or television meteorologist) and those who were nearby at the time may provide important information.

Low-Voltage Electrocution

Fatal electrocution from common household current often leaves no marks on its victim, and the autopsy gives no clues as to the cause of death. Consequently, low-voltage electrocution emphasizes the importance of a complete investigation to establish the cause and manner of death.

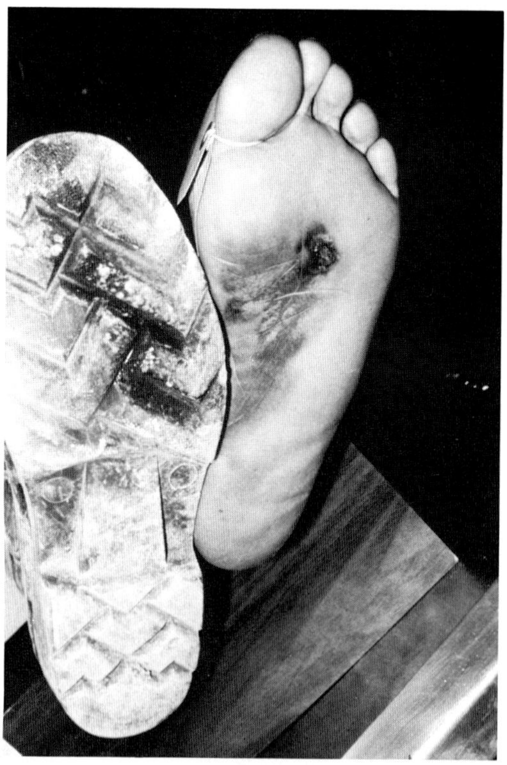

Figure 2.64 The shoe and foot are charred and indicate the points of electrical exit from a lightning strike on a golf course.

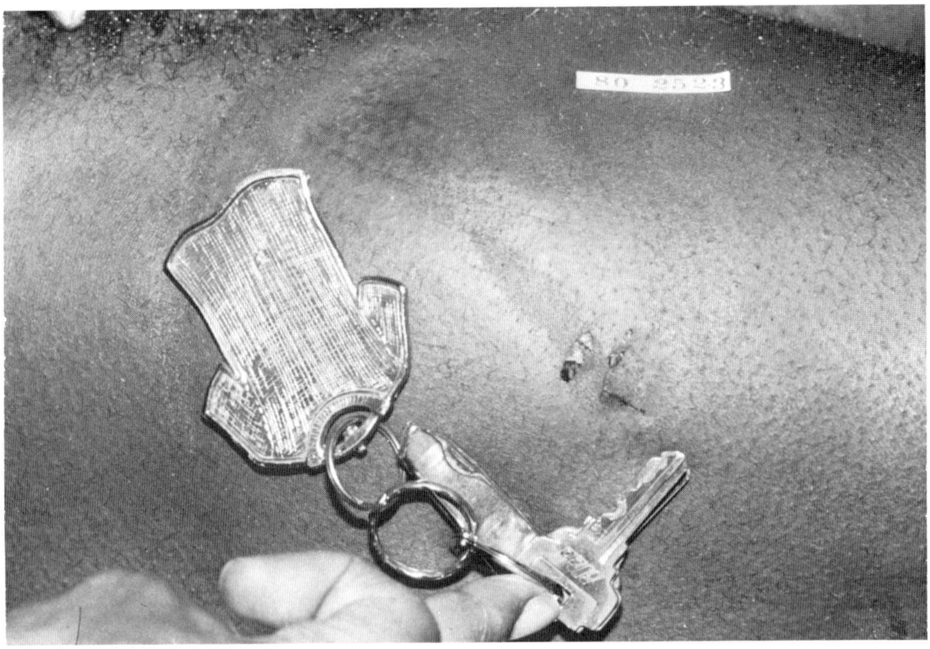

Figure 2.65 This skin burn resulted from contact with the keys as electrical energy was converted to thermal energy during a lightning strike.

Low-voltage electrocution should be suspected whenever death occurs near or during the operation of an electrical device. Suspicion is especially necessary whenever the electrical appliance is known to be defective (e.g., a "shocky lamp"). Electrical injury should also be ruled out in any case where the cause of death has not been determined after apparently adequate investigation. Since electrical burns are not expected in over 40% of the cases, and since low-voltage electrocution does not immediately incapacitate a person, electrocution should always be considered as a "rule-out diagnosis." In fact, a person sustaining fatal electrical injury has about 15 sec of consciousness and activity remaining before collapsing from ventricular fibrillation. During this time, the person may move, talk, shout, and even switch off or unplug the offending appliance.

Electrical burns are usually seen when the victim has prolonged contact with the offending tool or appliance after becoming incapacitated (Fig. 2.66). The autopsy findings, other than for electrical burns, should be expected to be non-revealing. Toxicological analyses of autopsy specimens should still be pursued to assist in excluding any contributory reckless behavior by the victim.

The appliance suspected of being electrically faulty must also be "autopsied." First inspect the appliance and all attached cords. Photograph anything abnormal. The appliance is then tested with a voltohmmeter as follows: With the voltohmmeter set at infinity, the prongs of the plug should be tested with the appliance in the on and off positions. A continuity of current should be

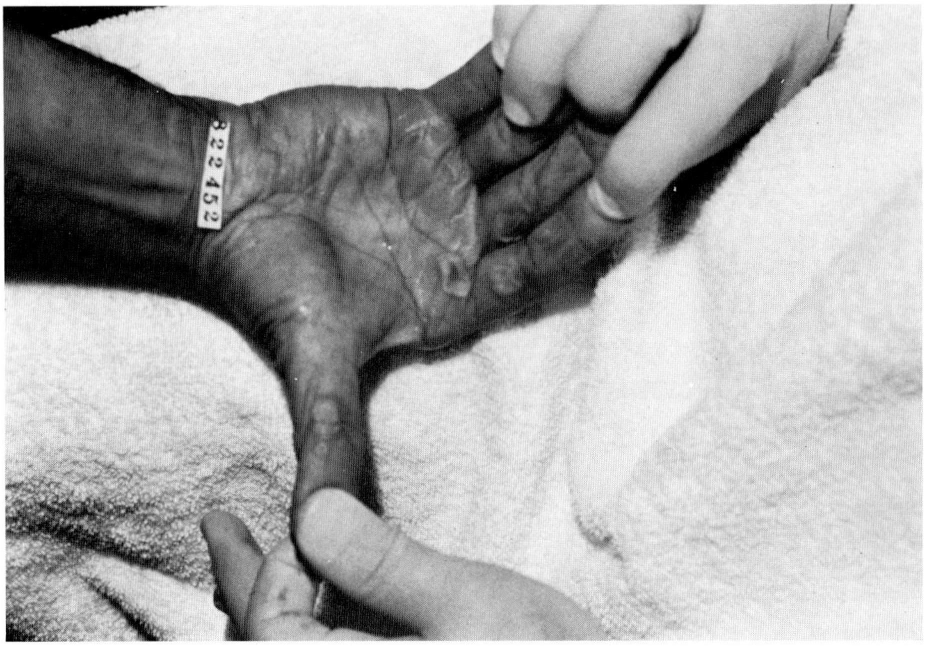

Figure 2.66 Electrical burns from prolonged contact with an energized hand tool (low-voltage electrocution).

evident. It is important to remember that the device should not be plugged into an electrical outlet during testing (unless the examiner would like to join the victim). Next, one prong is placed on the casing and the other on a prong of the plug. Any reading that implies that the casing is electrified indicates that a wire is in contact with the casing.

In most instances, disassembly of the suspect device is indicated. Photography of the disassembly, step by step, is important. Tool marks on screws connecting the casing together should also be noted and photographed, since they may indicate previous repairs by the owner or repair service. An eye toward civil litigation must also be maintained by the medical examiner, since the family may wish to sue the manufacturer or the repair service. If expert witnesses are hired by the plaintiff or the defense, it is best that the device be examined in the presence of the medical examiner to prevent any allegation of impropriety.

The outlet into which the appliance was plugged should also be checked with a circuit tester. This inexpensive device is simply plugged into the outlet, and the pattern of colored lights on the device indicates if the wiring is correct, if the ground is faulty, if there is a hot-neutral reverse, etc.

In some instances, it may be necessary actually to inspect the electrical wiring of a circuit box (this is usually best done by an electrician). Amateur dabblers in electrical repair may connect an independent wiring system to the electrical out-box, and therefore the main electrical switch may not cut off all the power. Unfortunate discoveries of such hazards are often made by the same person who installed the additional wiring in previous years: before making a repair in the attic or while installing a new ceiling fixture, he forgets that the main "switch off" lever will not turn off the current in the additional circuitry on which he is working.

Appendix: Using the Voltohmmeter to Test for Electrical Defects

The voltohmmeter (VOM) is an inexpensive instrument that can be used to test most electrical hand tools for evidence of an electrical defect. The device measures electrical resistance and registers readings between ∞ and 0 ohms. It operates by utilizing two independent probes, each of which is separately inserted into the VOM. Of course, when the two metal probes are touched together, the VOM scale will register 0 ohms because electricity is flowing freely through

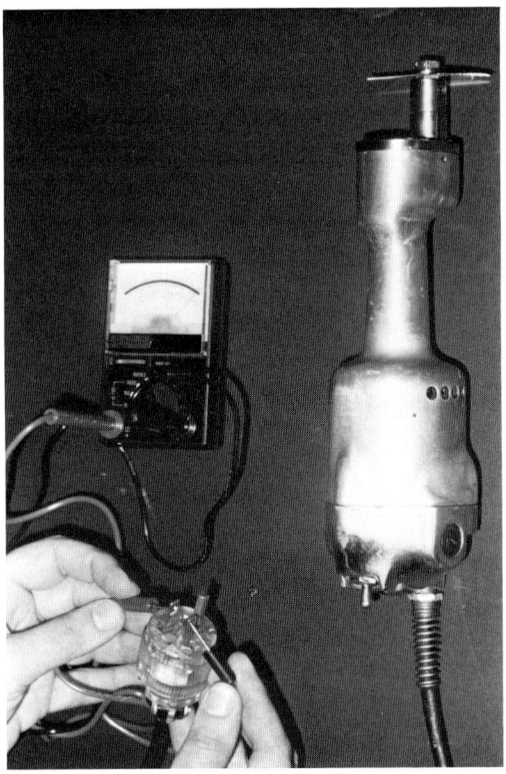

Figure 2.67 When each probe is touching one of the two current-carrying prongs, the VOM should register "0 ohms" (i.e., free current flow).

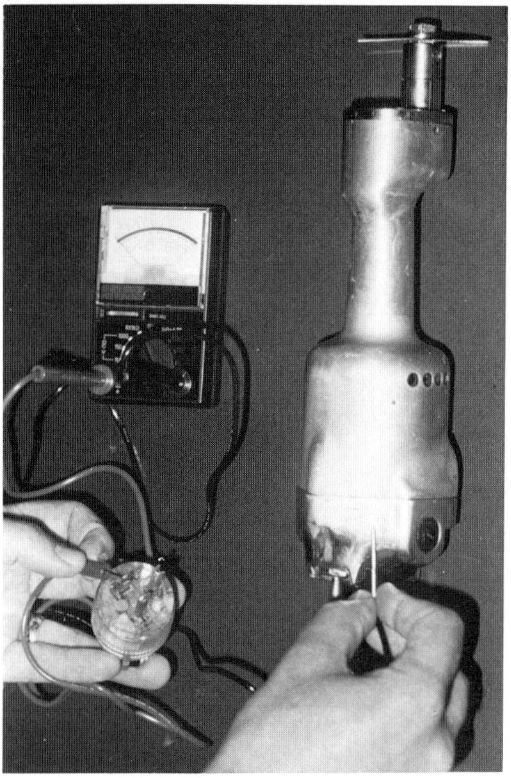

Figure 2.68 With one probe on a current-carrying prong and the other on the casing, the VOM should register ∞ ohms (i.e., no current flow). Any reading implies a short circuit. Both prongs should be similarly tested.

both wires and in through the machine, resulting in a complete circuit. When the probes are separated, no current can flow, and hence the machine will register ∞ ohms. These principles are used to check the casing of a suspect tool. When current flows into the tool through one prong, no current should register on the VOM when the second probe touches the casing. If it does, that implies that there is faulty electrical wiring making contact with the casing, which may permit electrocution. Thus, a machine may be tested as shown below with the switch in the "on" position (and the device unplugged).

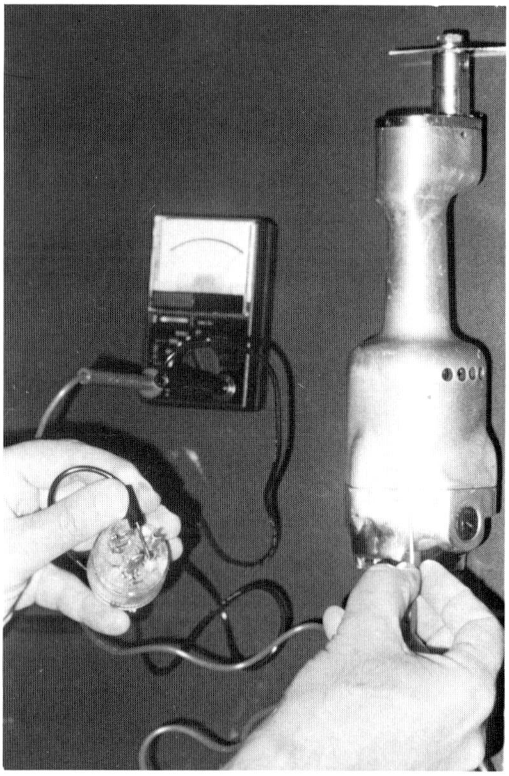

Figure 2.69 With one probe on the ground plug and the other on the case, the VOM should read 0 ohms (free current flow). This is expected, since the ground wire is directly connected to the casing. The ground wire is designed to provide safe passage of electricity if the casing should become energized. After the VOM readings are obtained and recorded, the device should be carefully opened, "autopsied," and photographed. The aberrant wire (making contact with the casing) is usually obvious.

DRUG OVERDOSE

Drug overdose is often not suspected at the scene of death, particularly when there is historical or physical evidence of a serious natural disease. However, we live in a drug- and alcohol-oriented society, and it must be remembered that just because a person has a natural disease, that disease is not necessarily the cause of death. People with cancer or heart disease do commit suicide with pills, and epileptics have been known to snort cocaine (an epileptogenic drug). Therefore, suspicion is the first step in diagnosis, regardless of the medical history.

Every death scene, particularly of apparently natural death, should be evaluated for the presence of drugs and alcohol. Ideally, all medication containers should be sent to the morgue with the body. These should then be checked as to date and amount issued, and the frequency with which they should have been taken. An empty bottle of digitalis or an antidepressant found at a death scene with yesterday's date has obvious implications. All recreational drug paraphernalia found at a death scene should also accompany the body to the morgue.

Aside from scene and historical evidence for an overdose of prescribed medication, external examination may also be suggestive. Specifically look for scars of the wrist, neck, and antecubital fossae suggestive of prior suicide attempts. Green, pink, or red stains of the mouth (skin, tongue, and between the teeth) or hands are suggestive of medication dye. Vomitus in or around the mouth may be similarly stained. At autopsy, be cognizant of any peculiar odors or gastrointestinal stains (usually bright green or red). In barbiturate overdoses, the gastric fundus is often hyperemic and has accentuated vascular markings. Save the entire gastric and small intestinal contents for quantification of ingested but unabsorbed medication. On the average (and this is a rule of thumb only), the equivalent of eight to ten pills remaining in the stomach is typical for suicidal overdose, whereas one or two pills is more typical of accidental overdose. Regardless of the suspected or identified medication, always check the blood for alcohol because of its potentiating (synergistic) effects. Death occurs at lower blood concentrations of drugs if alcohol or other depressant drugs are also ingested.

When the blood concentrations of drugs and/or alcohol are low, consider the possibility of positional or postural asphyxia. This occurs when the intoxicated individual passes out in a position resulting in partial airway obstruction (e.g., falling face down into a soft pillow, or lying with the head off the mattress and the body prone). Death results from a combination of hypoxia and the anesthetic effects of the alcohol and drugs. The process, however, may take hours, and during this time the substances are being metabolized or otherwise eliminated. To make the diagnosis, one must know the exact position of the body when found and carefully interpret the toxicologic results.

Suspicion of recreational drug overdose will depend on the social background of the individual and knowledge of what drugs are prevalent in a given community. Always remember that a death scene from recreational drug abuse is frequently cleaned up before the police are called: drugs and paraphernalia are removed to avoid guilt by association. External examination should include special attention to the following:

1. Nasal septum and nares should be checked for presence of white powdery material (e.g., cocaine) and ulcers, perforations, or inflammation (suggestive of chronic nasal insufflation).
2. Recent or old injection sites on upper extremities or other sites of predilection should be noted. High-profile individuals or those subject to frequent inspection (e.g., military personnel) may use small-gauge needles, rotate injection sites, or inject beneath a watch band. Consequently, recent injection sites may be imperceptible. If intravenous drug abuse is strongly suspected, incise areas of predilection that may

disclose the injection site (especially the antecubital fossa). If CPR was initiated, some of these sites may be iatrogenic and therefore render interpretation difficult.

3. Tattoos suggestive of a drug culture orientation should be noted (e.g., "Mr. Zigzag," the number 13 for "M," which stands for marijuana). Multiple tattoos of the upper extremities sometimes hide (or try to hide) old needle track scars.
4. Atrophic or circular scars of the upper extremities should be noted, as these may have been the site of previous injections (especially of cocaine). Chronic cutaneous ulcers or necrotizing fasciitis has a similar significance.
5. Bitemarks on the tongue, lips, or cheeks may suggest terminal seizures from an overdose with cocaine or amphetamine.
6. Frothy pulmonary edema fluid in the nose and mouth may be blood-tinged and may be dried over the nose and mouth. This is most typical for narcotic overdose, but may also be seen with cocaine and other drugs.

Intravenous drug abusers often have enlarged lymph nodes in the porta hepatis or around the celiac axis, and these should be specifically examined. Histologic sections should be taken of fresh, recent, and old injection sites, and of the lungs to look for granulomas and polarizable foreign materials (especially talc and starch). These result from the injection of oral medications, which frequently contain talc or starch or diluents. A section of the liver should be taken to check for the presence of viral hepatitis. Also examine the spleen for accentuation of the white pulp common among intravenous narcotic users.

Toxicologic specimens to be taken in all cases of suspected drug overdose include:

all ocular fluid;
50 ml blood in sodium flouride;
10 ml blood in sodium fluoride (as "retainer tube");
300 gm liver;
10 ml bile;
50 ml urine (or all available up to 50 ml);
stomach contents and small bowel contents, particularly in the case of suspected medication overdose.

The bile and liver are particularly helpful to obtain the ratio of parent drug to its primary metabolite. This may help in the evaluation of acute or chronic ingestion of a substance. Also, it may identify a case as an accidental overdose when the concentration of the parent compound is low but the longer-lived pharmacologically active metabolite is in a high concentration (e.g., propoxyphene and norproproxyphene).

Keep in mind that someone who supplies a controlled substance that results in death may be charged with a felony murder, depending on how the law is worded. A legal identification and strict observance of the chain of custody of the toxicologic specimens may therefore be warranted in some cases.

CHILDHOOD DEATHS

Infanticide

Suspicion of infanticide usually begins when a baby, with or without the placenta, is found unceremoniously disposed of, or when the mother presents to an emergency room with vaginal bleeding and denies a recent pregnancy despite physical signs to the contrary. The responsibility of the pathologist is to provide evidence that the infant did in fact sustain an extrauterine existence, no matter how brief. (If the death occurred *in utero* due to actions of the mother or another person, the case would be prosecuted under the criminal abortion statutes, not the homicide statutes.)

All measurements should be carefully made to establish if the fetus had attained an age of viability. Roentgenograms that indicate aeration of the lungs and gastrointestinal tract should be retained. The autopsy should be directed at documenting a live birth: aeration of lungs, air in the stomach, swallowed extrauterine materials, etc. If the child was "delivered" into a toilet bowl, it may well have swallowed water and blood. Check the blood for fetal hemoglobin. Also look for neck injuries and interpret these carefully: they may represent strangulation or may have been caused by the mother attempting to extricate the baby. Be sure to include infection of the fetus or placenta, which might be a source of gas formation and "aerated lungs."

Be sure to inform the police not to ask leading questions regarding attempts to "save a blue baby." Blowing air into an infant's face will aerate the lungs and gastrointestinal tract, thus obscuring any evidence of live birth.

Since smothering is a frequent cause of death in these cases, the main value of the autopsy (besides ascertaining a live birth) is to exclude other causes of death. Nonetheless, look for conjunctival petechiae and for mouth injuries (particulary a torn frenulum) that would be consistent with smothering.

Child Abuse

Children who are not chronically abused but who die from a single injury delivered by a parent or surrogate parent are more aptly designated childhood homicides. These children have no evidence of prior physical abuse and the case is handled in much the same way as an adult homicide. The major problem for the pathologist is to determine if the purported "accident" is consistent with the observed injuries and the developmental capabilities of the child.

Children with evidence of chronic abuse usually succumb to one or more acute injuries such as a blow to the head or abdomen, or the whiplash shaken infant syndrome. The fatal injuries should be clearly separated from those indicative of repetitive injuries. The reason is that the perpetrator may be accused only of administering a fatal injury and not aggravated child abuse. In this circumstance, the mention of prior injuries during a trial may well be deemed prejudicial to a jury and lead to a mistrial.

Sometimes a child dies from the cumulative result of repeated injuries (with or without food deprivation), and a single fatal injury cannot be identified. In this circumstance we have found it best to list the cause of death simply as "child abuse syndrome."

All children below the age of 6 years should have total body X-rays, particularly those suspected of death from child abuse or childhood homicide. If necessary, obtain the consultation of a radiologist to determine the time frame when fractures would have occurred, their stage of healing, and for the detection of other, subtle changes consistent with maltreatment.

Always examine and photograph the frenulum (Fig. 2.70). An injury here is usually indicative of a punch or slap, jamming a bottle into the mouth, or a shearing stress applied when the nose is pinched and the mouth covered (while trying to silence a crying infant). All patterned injuries must be thoroughly photographed. After all the obvious has been recorded and photographed (including the frenulum), stand back and specifically look for minor abrasions and bruises, particularly of the back, shoulders, and arms (fingertip bruises from shaking the child) and the buttocks (severe spanking). These areas should be carefully incised and, if bruising is detected, histologic sections should be taken. Next, specifically look at the genitalia for evidence of sexual abuse. In males, look for pinch marks of the scrotum and for injuries consistent with ligatures being applied to the penis.

All internal injuries should be approached with the idea of establishing when the injury occurred insofar as possible. This may be particularly difficult but important with abdominal injuries, when there may be a delay between the infliction of the injury and the actual death. Also note what injuries are or are not consistent with CPR (often invoked as a cause for the rib fractures or hepatic injury).

After evisceration, dry the body cavities and carefully examine for rib fractures. Histologically document the varying stages of healing (fresh fractures to old callous formations). Do the same for any extremity fractures or periosteal elevations initially detected radiologically.

Photograph the reflected scalp and exposed skull whether or not there are any injuries. Again, look for fingertip bruises. If subdural or subarachnoid blood is detected, the whiplash shaken infant syndrome should be suspected—especially if there is no skull fracture. Remove the eyes and fix in formalin before making

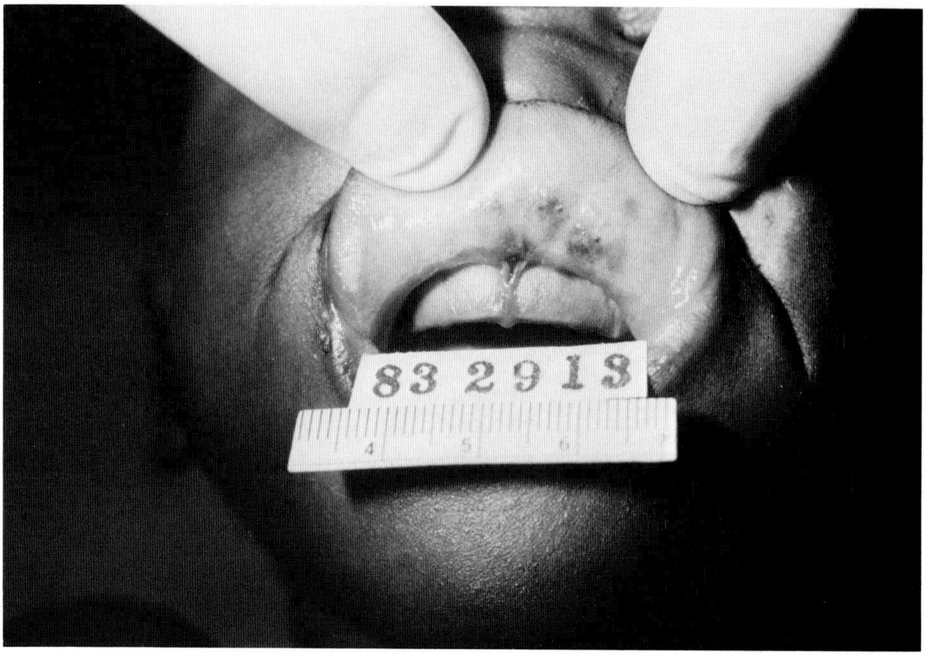

Figure 2.70 A laceration to the frenulum is an indicator of child abuse "until proven otherwise." This structure must be examined in every infant and childhood death.

histologic sections to demonstrate extravasated blood in the retina. Photograph the interior of the skull after removing the dura mater.

Once the autopsy is complete, rephotograph the body after overnight refrigeration. Frequently, bruises not evident on the initial examination will appear.

In the case of death due to neglect and starvation, the effort should be directed to establishing the developmental age of the child and contrasting that with observed physical characteristics (such as weight, length, etc.). The developmental age must be established by historical data (birth date), histologic changes, and radiologic evaluation (bone age).

The second area of importance is to exclude, insofar as possible, the presence of any underlying congenital defect that could account for a failure to thrive. Particular attention must therefore be given to measurements of physical characteristics, the amount of subcutaneous and body fat, and to histologic sampling (especially the immune system and gastrointestinal tract).

Deaths from scalding should clearly document all immersion lines both diagrammatically and photographically. Also, the child should be positioned to demonstrate leg or body flexion to account for the scalding pattern and the intervening area not scalded (protected by flexed legs, etc.).

Toxicologic testing is usually not done in child abuse fatalities unless there is some evidence that the child was chronically given alcohol or antihistamines to provide continuous sedation. This information may surface at a subsequent date. Hence, a fluoride-preserved blood sample should be retained.

Crib Death

The diagnosis of the sudden infant death syndrome (SIDS) is one of exclusion, both at the scene and at the autopsy. The usual scenario is that the mother feeds the child, puts it to sleep, and a few hours later finds the child dead. A small amount of bloody fluid may be in or around the mouth, depending on the position of the child. At times, lividity on one of the cheeks is interpreted by the discovering parent as a bruise. A history of premature birth and low socioeconomic status is frequent. The child is usually between 2 weeks and 6 months of age. In our experience, SIDS is quite rare beyond 6 months of age.

The postmortem examination is ''negative.'' No significant abnormalities are observed externally (except, perhaps, for a diaper rash). Radiologic examination is also negative. The internal examination is devoid of any findings apart from petechiae of the thymus, epicardium, pleuras, and visceral congestion. The stomach usually contains some food remnants (curdled milk is most typical). Blood cultures are usually negative. If positive, they are quite difficult to interpret when no infection is apparent. In general, approach the autopsy to specifically exclude natural disease, congenital anomaly, and childhood homicide. Remember that the findings in a smothered baby may be identical with those of SIDS.

It is recommended that tissue samples of the following be obtained for histologic review: cerebral cortex (to rule out an early meningitis or unsuspected encephalitis), epiglottis, trachea, submandibular salivary gland (for viral inclusions), thyroid, lung, heart, liver, pancreas, spleen, and kidneys. A fluoride-preserved blood sample should be obtained for possible toxicologic testing.

If the scene, circumstances, and gross autopsy findings are typical for SIDS, the death certificate is completed immediately. A letter is sent to the parents explaining what SIDS is, that it cannot be predicted, and that it cannot be prevented. This helps alleviate parental anxiety and allay the suspicions of other family members or neighbors. Ideally, a visiting nurse or public health official subsequently visits the family to ensure their understanding, avert unfounded accusations of neglect that may be directed to one or both parents, and answer any questions about SIDS.

Occasionally, one discovers an unexpected myocarditis or other process upon subsequent histologic examination. In that case, the death certificate is amended and an appropriate followup is afforded to the parents. Since this is really an ''explained SIDS'', nothing has been lost by the letter sent to the parents (and the nurse's visit). Invariably, the myocarditis or other problem would, for all practical purposes, have been virtually impossible to predict or prevent. Since more good than harm results from this approach, it is better to err in favor of relieving guilt and recrimination than to allow parental anxiety to proceed needlessly for the sake of academic accuracy.

CHAPTER 3

Special Problems

INTRODUCTION

Special problems arise in certain cases and situations because they require more investigation than is usual, and because they have the most potential for serious error. The most troublesome cases are usually those in which the identification of the victim or the cause of death is unknown or uncertain. The most troublesome situations are those that tend to overwhelm the system by the large number of cases involved (mass disaster), or because the case has evoked intense community interest (the high-profile case). The special problem case requires close attention to detail and resistance to pressures to prematurely finalize or release the case. Above all, it is necessary to prepare a detailed plan of action and interagency coordination before the high-profile case or situation actually arises.

NO IDENTIFICATION

In most instances, an unknown decedent is identified fairly quickly by police agencies. Fingerprints and missing persons reports are perhaps the most frequent tools utilized by the police. Also helpful are Polaroid photographs of the deceased that are shown to local residents as police do their area canvass. When fingerprints and visual identification are not possible (decomposed bodies, fire deaths, etc.), the identification is usually presumptive and subsequently confirmed by dental record comparison or other means (comparing postmortem with antemortem X-rays, etc.). In a small percentage of cases, however, these routine procedures fail to disclose the identity of a person. This frequently occurs because the decedent had not established any social ties within the community, as is common with drifters, newly arrived immigrants, and homicide victims whose bodies are transported elsewhere and discarded. Since the law does not usually specify who has the primary responsibility for identifying a deceased person, the responsibility is generally shared by both the police and the medical examiner. The main job of the medical examiner is to provide as much information as possible to the police. The police then utilize this information at the local, state, and federal levels in an attempt to establish a presumptive identification that will eventually lead to confirmed identity.

In some instances, all efforts fail to reveal an identity, and the deceased must simply be buried as an unknown. This, however, should never be done until all possible information about the body is satisfactorily obtained and preserved.

Once the fingerprints and facial photographs have been taken, and the identity of the victim remains unknown, proceed with the following steps:

1. Carefully inspect and diagram the body, making particular note of general features (hair and eye color, weight, stature, approximate age, etc.) as well as specific characteristics (scars, tattoos, prostheses, etc.).
2. Take detailed photographs of the entire body.
3. Record and photograph all clothing and jewelry. Pay particular attention to labels, size, style, laundry markings, etc. on the clothing, and look for inscriptions on the jewelry. Be sure to turn all pockets inside out or, if necessary, cut the clothing to completely expose the contents of the pockets.
4. Photograph and chart the teeth. This usually requires the help of a dentist. If possible, dental X-rays should be taken, and one should also consider taking dental impressions. If none of this is possible or feasible, and the body is decomposed or charred from a fire, simply remove and skeletonize the upper and lower jaws.
5. Take full body X-rays. Be sure these are of good enough quality to permit their comparison with antemortem X-rays should they become available.
6. Make specific notes about any possible medical conditions uncovered by the autopsy, particularly of any operative procedures (appendectomy, hysterectomy, etc.).

The information should be given to the police, and a National Crime Information Center (NCIC) form should be completed and submitted as well. The NCIC form may be obtained from the police. These forms, along with procedures and diagrams, are also available in the College of American Pathologists (CAP) *Handbook for Postmortem Examination of Undetermined Remains*. At this point, the police and/or medical examiner should enlist the help of the local news media. Although usually cooperative, they may have a policy of not showing a photograph of a dead person's face. They will, however, show a sketch made by a police artist as well as photographs of clothing and jewelry.

NO CAUSE OF DEATH

Under certain circumstances, it is expected that the postmortem examination will not reveal an apparent cause of death, or may only disclose mild and nonspecific abnormalities. These include the sudden infant death syndrome, many cases of drug overdose, death from environmental exposure, and sudden death in individuals with a history of epilepsy, asthma, or "functional" cardiovascular diseases (e.g., Romano-Ward syndrome). Such cases do not present much of a problem, since the combination of histologic, toxicologic, and, particularly, historical and medical data allows one to reasonably conclude the cause of death. However, the "negative autopsy" is a real problem when sudden death occurs in the absence of any medical history or when there is no suspicion that the death was related to drugs or poisons. In this circumstance, four possibilities should be considered: (1) that something major was overlooked at the scene (or the scene was "cleaned up" before the police arrived—particularly likely for drug overdose cases); (2) that something was missed at the autopsy table; (3) that toxicologic analysis, chemical testing, or histologic examination will reveal the cause of death; (4) that the history (medical, social, or terminal event) is erroneous or incomplete.

The realization that you have a "negative autopsy," and no realistic suspicion as to a cause of death, usually occurs at the autopsy table. At that point, reexamine the organs you have already removed and dissected. Look specifically at the orifices to the coronary arteries (sometimes the only atherosclerotic plaque in the body encroaches one orifice), review the coronary arteries again (regardless of age), and examine the mitral valve for redundancy and myxomatous changes. Check the pulmonary vasculature for thromboemboli and for atherosclerotic changes indicative of pulmonary hypertension. Examine the bronchi and lungs for possible evidence of asthmatic bronchitis. Remove the tongue and serially section to detect any hemorrhagic foci consistent with bitemarks from terminal seizures. Inspect the lips and cheeks for the same purpose. Visualize (if possible) and palpate the hypopharynx and posterior nasopharynx for a foreign object or chunk of food that may have obstructed the airway and subsequently become dislodged. Incise the antecubital fossae for occult intravenous injection sites, and inspect the area of the wrist normally covered by a watch band for the same purpose. If all this is nonrevealing, save the entire heart and the brain in formaldehyde, take multiple histologic sections, and be sure you have taken enough fluid and tissue for toxicologic testing (include tests for heavy metals, carbon monoxide, and cyanide). Acetone should also be tested for, since its presence may indicate a previously unsuspected diabetic ketoacidosis. Submit the ocular fluid sample (with no preservative) for glucose, urea nitrogen, creatinine, and electrolyte determinations. At this point, one must sign the death certificate as "undetermined, pending further investigation." If the victim had been transported to a hospital emergency room, be sure to obtain the paramedical rescue report, the emergency room records, and any blood, urine, or gastric lavage specimens they may have.

The next step, which should be done as soon as possible after the autopsy is completed, is to eliminate subtle environmental causes of death. This may require the aid of the police. Confirm the exact position of the body when it was initially discovered. Determine if the death could have resulted from household electrocution (after low-voltage electric shock, the person may unplug and put away an appliance before collapsing with ventricular fibrillation). Also determine if there is a possible source of carbon monoxide (e.g., air conditioning intake placed inside a garage), since deaths from low levels of carbon monoxide (as may occur in people with chronic lung disease) may not result in a color change of the blood or musculature. Finally, insofar as possible, ascertain whether the death could have been the result of food aspiration (the food having been removed by witnesses or rescue personnel) or drug overdose (bottles or paraphernalia having been removed by whoever discovered the body).

Finally, one must resort to the most important investigative tool of all, the telephone. Personally talk with all physicians who had contact with the decedent during life, obtain all medical records, and talk with as many family members or acquaintances as possible. The idea here is to obtain any clinical indication of an occult cardiovascular or central nervous system disorder. Consequently, questions about seizures, syncope, shortness of breath, chest pain, and related topics are necessary. Also inquire about the habits of the deceased, childhood illnesses, and the health and causes of death of family members.

When the histologic sections arrive, look specifically for natural processes associated with sudden death: myocarditis (which may be patchy and fairly subtle), primary pulmonary hypertension, asthmatic bronchitis, diabetes mellitus, etc. Finally, after as much data as possible has been accumulated, one must decide whether to add additional histologic sections, expand the toxicologic analysis, or obtain consultants in cardiac pathology and neuropathology.

Sudden death and a "negative autopsy" is often the most challenging case faced by a medical examiner. Usually these turn out to be natural deaths, and the diagnosis is established by a combination of historical and histologic evidence. The very nature of these cases also means that the diagnosis is frequently based on a "preponderance of evidence" rather than the more comfortable degree of certainty afforded by "reasonable medical probability."

Summary

I. At the Autopsy Table:

1. Review all organs.
   —check coronary artery orifices, coronary arteries, mitral valve.
   —check for pulmonary thromboemboli.
   —examine for bitemarks (tongue, lips, cheeks).

—visualize and palpate hypopharynx and posterior nasopharynx for foreign objects.

2. Make incisions to uncover occult needle marks.
3. Obtain full toxicologic analysis (include acetone, carbon monoxide, cyanide, and heavy metals).
4. Determine urea nitrogen, creatinine, glucose, and electrolytes in ocular fluid.
5. Take multiple histologic sections.
6. Preserve heart and brain in formaldehyde.

II. Immediately After the Autopsy:

1. Obtain report of paramedical rescue units, emergency room records, and any specimens taken by emergency room personnel if these were not already requested.
2. Inspect clothing (especially pockets) of deceased. (If the clothes were taken by the hospital emergency room or the police, obtain them and do not assume they have already been inspected.)
3. Be sure the scene investigation addressed the possibilities of household electrocution, positional asphyxia, drug overdose, occult source of carbon monoxide, food or foreign object aspiration, and toxic environmental exposure.

III. Soon After the Autopsy:

1. Obtain copies of all medical records.
2. Consult with all physicians who treated or examined the deceased during life.
3. Converse with as many family members and acquaintances of the deceased as possible regarding health and habits.

IV. Obtain Necessary Pathologist Consultation:

1. Cardiac pathologist.
2. Neuropathologist.

ENVIRONMENTAL EXPOSURE

Fatalities due to hypothermia or hyperthermia are determined mainly by the circumstances of death and the conditions under which the body is discovered. The autopsy findings are generally nonspecific but nevertheless assist in uncovering contributory factors and excluding other causes of death. The workup for both types of thermal deaths is essentially the same:

1. Determination of environmental conditions (e.g., temperature, humidity, wind chill factor, dampness, ventilation of room).

2. Length of exposure time to thermal conditions.
3. Presence and condition of clothing (e.g., wet, moist, dry), evidence of paradoxical undressing as seen with deaths from hypothermia.
4. Determination of risk factors.
   A. Elderly, infant, poor physical condition, medical illness or injury, obesity, senility.
   B. Alcoholism.
   C. Degree of physical activity.
   D. Lack of acclimatization.
5. Autopsy
   A. Toxicology: ethanol and other drugs.
   B. Exclude other causes of death (natural causation).
   C. Vitreous humor electrolyte determinations for evidence of dehydration.

Hyperthermic deaths may well be associated with an elevated postmortem body temperature even hours after death. A core temperature may be taken by inserting a thermometer deep into the liver or brain. A hypothermic death is more difficult to document by postmortem temperature readings, since it is usually unknown how long the person has been dead. Finally one must consider the role of environmental exposure in accelerating the death of a person with underlying natural disease, particularly the elderly. If there is reasonable suspicion that exposure contributed to the death, then the immediate cause of death should be listed as the underlying disease (e.g., arteriosclerotic heart disease) and the exposure as a contributory cause of death. The manner of death, then, would be accidental.

The autopsy is usually nonspecific despite claims of pathologic findings in various organs. External examination may reveal localized thermal injuries (e.g., sunburn, frostbite) suggesting environmental exposure, but this is usually not enough to finalize an opinion. Bright pink lividity may be encountered in people dying from hypothermia. Although this has been attributed to the postmortem diffusion of oxygenated blood into the skin, the same phenomenon occurs in those who are known to die of natural causes and whose body is subsequently frozen (e.g., on cruise ships).

Unfortunately there is no magical formula to determine whether or not death was due to thermal cause. The investigator must correlate environmental conditions with the terminal circumstances of death, the medical history, and the autopsy to form a satisfactory conclusion. In the vast majority of cases, death from environmental exposure is regarded as accidental. However, homicide should be considered in exposure deaths involving children or the elderly. It is also conceivable that suicide may be the appropriate manner of death in some mentally deranged persons.

Checklist for Environmental Exposure Deaths

1. Scene visit.
   A. Determine environmental temperature, humidity, and air convection on day of death as well as several days prior to the death.
   B. Location of body.
      1. Outdoors or indoors? If indoors, check the function of heaters or air conditioners as appropriate. If cold outdoors, look for evidence of paradoxical undressing.
      2. Localized moisture near body (e.g., body in water, wet clothes).
2. Identification of decedent.
3. Length of exposure time (if known).
4. Medical history of decedent.
5. Terminal circumstances of life (e.g., physical activity).
6. Autopsy.
   A. Pink-red lividity.
   B. Localized injuries of frostbite or sunburn.
   C. Other causes of death, and natural diseases that could make a person more susceptible to exposure.
7. Toxicology: alcohol, antidepressants, psychotropic medications; if hyperthermia is suspected, test for cocaine and amphetamines.

THE DECOMPOSED BODY

By its very nature, the body in moderate to advanced stages of decomposition poses numerous problems. Unless it is an obvious homicide,scene investigation is often less than thorough due to the repugnant odors, particularly if the body is inside a domicile and the scene investigators are not experienced with this situation. For similar reasons, the autopsy itself may be less than thorough, depending on the experience, tolerance, and interest of the pathologist. Despite the repugnant nature of these cases, it is imperative that the scene investigation and the autopsy itself be approached with even more care and attention to detail than for the nondecomposed body. This is because the process of decomposition destroys anatomical changes that would otherwise be obvious, and it creates artifacts that hinder accurate interpretation. Hence, relatively subtle changes become more significant in the attempt to establish a cause of death. Even with a thorough scene investigation and a nonhurried, carefully performed autopsy, all phases of the death investigation are severely encumbered, especially identification, the significance of the autopsy findings, and toxicologic analysis.

For obvious reasons, visual identification of the deceased is usually not possible and greater reliance is placed on circumstantial identification, particularly when there is no reasonable suspicion of homicide. However, when greater assurance of identification is needed, fingerprints may still be obtained even in advanced stages of decomposition. Often the superficial epidermal layer (with the fingerprint ridges) will separate, and this layer can be removed like a glove and given to the crime laboratory. In other instances, the fingers must be cut off individually and submitted to the laboratory. Naturally, one may also rely on dental and radiologic features for purposes of identification. In some instances it may be advisable to remove and preserve the mandible and maxilla for future dental comparisons.

If the process of decomposition is predominantly that of mummification or of adipocere formation, full body X-rays should be taken. The major reason for this is to locate any projectiles or foreign objects, since these modes of decomposition often obscure external injuries that would otherwise be obvious. Putrefactive decomposition, on the other hand, usually (but not always) accentuates external injuries because of the gas formation. The accentuated injury is often accompanied by marked distortion and also appears as a focus of decomposition somewhat more advanced than the remainder of the body. These areas should be radiologically evaluated. Incidentally, recent surgical scars also break down more rapidly and may therefore be initially confused with a recent injury. Usually, suture material can be identified in the depths of the defect.

The autopsy technique is also modified in decomposed bodies that cannot be viewed at a funeral home. The midline autopsy incision is made to extend from the mental symphysis to the pubic symphysis. The interacromion incision remains the same. This enables the pathologist to more easily expose the neck structures and lessens the chance of creating artifactual fractures. Also, facial and extremity incisions are often needed to discover contusions not otherwise visible because of the distortion and discoloration.

Toxicologic analysis is hampered both by the lack of fluids and tissues and by interference with the testing itself by decomposition products. Very often, blood, urine, bile, ocular fluid, and gastric contents have totally disappeared. One is then limited to obtaining decomposing chest fluid, brain, and liver (although other tissues, such as lung and kidney, may also be useful in some circumstances). Alcohol levels in both blood and brain are often spuriously elevated. In our experience, an alcohol concentration up to 0.10% (in decomposed chest fluid or brain) is attributed to putrefactive decomposition. Drug concentrations are generally not very meaningful and usually have more of a qualitative than a quantitative significance. Drug analysis should nonetheless be attempted when indicated. Even drugs that are rapidly metabolized and disintegrate in the postmortem state, such as cocaine, may still be detected in decomposed brain or chest fluid.

The autopsy findings in decomposed bodies are often meager, and frequently what is not found is more significant than what is found. Thus, in what appears to be a natural death, the only significant finding might be focal calcification of the coronary arteries, suggesting the death was due to arteriosclerotic heart disease. Of equal and perhaps greater significance was that there was also no evidence of a skull fracture, intracranial blood, fractured ribs, etc. Therefore, even though the apparent cause of death is not demonstrated to the greatest degree of satisfaction, at least an obviously traumatic death has been excluded. The following case is illustrative:

A moderately decomposed, 58-year-old man is found in a prone position on the living room floor. An upright vacuum cleaner (cord unplugged) is beside his body. The decedent was a retired, well-adjusted military officer who lived alone in his neat, well-ventilated home. The medical history was completely unremarkable and there was no history of substance abuse. The vacuum cleaner and electrical outlet in the wall were free of electrical defects. The home was locked, in order, and without evidence of a breakin.

The autopsy findings consisted of dark, moist lungs weighing 150 g each. The 450-g heart appeared slightly enlarged. The coronary arteries were calcific. However, the degree of arteriosclerosis could not be determined because of the decomposition. Some undeterminable degree of nephrosclerosis could be perceived. The aorta had moderate atherosclerosis. The stomach was free of drug residue. Postmortem toxicology was entirely negative.

Although the autopsy findings were not dramatic, the preponderance of evidence indicated this man died from a cardiac rhythm disturbance, probably the result of hypertensive cardiovascular disease. The rationale for this decision is based upon the following:

A. The scene findings do not suggest foul play (e.g., robbery), environmental danger (e.g., carbon monoxide), or other hazards (electrocution).
B. The scene findings suggest sudden collapse (i.e., about to begin vacuuming), typical for a cardiac dysrhythmia.
C. The autopsy findings are not those indicative of traumatic death but are consistent with natural disease process suggestive of arteriosclerotic and/or hypertensive cardiovascular disease (viz., cardiomegaly, nephrosclerosis, aortic atherosclerosis). The fact that organ weights decrease with progressive decomposition further supports the diagnosis of cardiomegaly in this case.
D. There is no evidence of drug overdose.

As this case illustrates, the manner of death is sometimes more apparent with decomposed bodies than is the cause of death. At times it may be necessary to leave the cause of death unclassified while nonetheless indicating the probable manner of death on the death certificate. Thus, when the decomposition is so advanced that a cause of death cannot be reasonably established by the autopsy, one must rely almost entirely on the scene investigation, medical history, and circumstances of death. The same rationale applies to "homicide by undetermined means":

The severely decomposed body of a 30-year-old woman was found under the crawl space of her apartment. The body was wrapped in bedsheets identical to the sheet upon the mattress within her apartment. Drag marks led from the entrance of the crawl space to where the body was deposited. The decedent's apartment had been cleaned and her clothes were gone. Her boyfriend claimed he had left town after an argument a few days prior to her disappearance.

The autopsy revealed nothing except advanced putrefactive decomposition. Toxicology was negative for the usual drugs of abuse. Dental records established the identification.

The decedent worked as a hotel maid and was considered a good worker. Her medical history was unremarkable and she did not drink or use drugs. She had, on more than one occasion, appeared at work with scratches on her neck stemming from altercations with her boyfriend. The scene of death, the available background information, and the action of the boyfriend all indicate that the probable manner of death is homicide. The only other reasonable hypothesis for the unceremonious disposal of a dead body in this fashion would be an accidental drug overdose. However, there was no evidence to support this contention. Although the cause of death was most likely some variant of mechanical asphyxiation, the postmortem examination could not demonstrate this. Consequently, the cause of death was simply stated as undetermined, and the probable manner of death was listed as homicide. Others prefer to list the cause of death in such cases as "homicide by undetermined means." Again, one must rely on the preponderance of evidence instead of reasonable medical probability as to the manner of death.

SKELETAL REMAINS

The endpoint of decomposition is, of course, skeletonization. The forensic problems associated with the discovery of skeletal remains are much the same as with bodies discovered in advanced stages of decomposition. However, the scene investigation must center about the recovery of all the skeletal remains and other evidence. The role of the pathologist is to first ascertain whether the remains are human, animal, or commingled (more than one human, or mixed human and animal). The next task is to determine age, race, sex, stature, and, if possible, the cause and manner of death. Finally, efforts are directed toward identification of the deceased.

Ideally, four consultants should be contacted upon the discovery of skeletal remains: a botanist, an entomologist, a forensic odontologist, and a physical anthropologist. The botanist, aware of the flora and climatic changes, is quite helpful in estimating the time of death. The entomologist is useful for the same purpose by identifying any residual insects or their larvae. The odontologist and anthropologist are helpful in determining physical characteristics and in the ultimate identification of the deceased. Obviously, most do not have the luxury of these specialists, but if available, they are of great help.

Crime scene investigators will generally photograph the scene, make an area canvass for other evidence, and arrange for aerial photographs to be taken. The skeleton, along with any attached clothing or other artifacts, should be removed as intact as possible. The soil for at least 12 inches around and 6 inches deep should be placed in a container and subsequently sifted through screen mesh (¼ inch and ⅛ inch in succession) to retrieve any teeth, bones, bullets, or other artifacts such as buttons or jewelry. The scene investigation becomes more complex when the skeletal remains are distributed over a wide area because of dismemberment, animal activity, or when the remains are discovered during land clearing for a construction project. After a careful area canvass and overall photography (ideally including aerial photographs as well), the entire area is roped off and envisioned like a grid or a checkerboard. The location of each bone or other piece of evidence is then mapped and photographed in place. When bones or other artifacts are found, the underlying soil in that grid square must be sifted through wire screens.

Upon arrival at the morgue, the remains are first radiographed with the clothing on to detect any foreign objects. The clothing and other artifacts are then removed, separately photographed, and inventoried. If necessary, X-ray the bones without the clothing to detect any abnormalities and bony peculiarities that could help in subsequent identification, and for the detection of metallic particles that might suggest a death from stabbing or a firearms injury. Next, the skeleton should be assembled, photographed extensively, and inspected for age, race, sex, stature, and identifying features (old fractures, evidence of bone disease, etc.). Close attention should be given to the skull, ribs, and vertebrae, since these frequently have evidence of stab and gunshot wounds as well as blunt force injury.

Any remaining flesh should be removed from the bones. A variety of methods have been used for this purpose, depending on the amount of flesh and the type of decomposition. Among the favorites are boiling in an ammonia solution, soaking in warm water and bleach, exposure to carnivorous insects, and soaking for several days in warm water with a meat tenderizer (which has papain as the active ingredient).

Much of the foregoing will depend on the experience, training, and expertise of the examining pathologist. Assuming the pathologist has had no experience or training in physical anthropology, the best approach is to concentrate on preserving evidence: clean, photograph, X-ray, and inspect for obvious injuries. The bones can then be shipped to a consulting anthropologist or medical examiner, or simply stored in a labeled cardboard box until the remains are identified.

Also, if there are no clues as to the identity, the medical examiner or police might consider more sophisticated techniques, such as facial reconstruction. The CAP *Handbook for Postmortem Examination of Unidentified Remains* has a listing of individuals skilled in facial reconstruction.

Solitary human bones often are discovered without the remainder of the skeleton. Usually these are skulls, and they may come from a variety of sources. Skulls with East Indian features, with springs connecting the jaws and clips to hold the calvarium in place, are usually from medical or dental schools. Wartime trophy skulls often have had the occipital base broken out so they could be used as lamps. And sometimes skulls are found in association with certain religious rituals. If these are not obviously former medical or dental school specimens, they may have been smuggled into the country, or they may have been obtained by grave robbing. One must also consider the possibility of a disrupted grave site (or a burial at sea), in which case the bones may have anthropological or archeological significance.

DEATHS IN POLICE CUSTODY AND POLICE SHOOTINGS

Deaths resulting from shooting by a law enforcement officer or occurring in police custody are two of the most high-profile investigations faced by a medical examiner. A death in police custody invariably leads to allegations of police neglect or police brutality (even torture). In a police shooting, the initial question is whether or not the use of lethal force was justified. However, regardless of the facts, the incident itself may spark community violence—a riot.

Both situations generate intense community interest. The news media, police commanders, prosecuting attorneys, local officials, and community leaders want and need as much accurate information as possible, and as soon as possible. All phases of the investigation, including the autopsy report, will be critically scrutinized by all those directly concerned with the investigation as well as the public at large. The pressure to provide immediate answers enhances the possibility of error and the potential for public criticism of any or all of the investigating parties. For the medical examiner, the ultimate charge would be that of participating in a police coverup. Consequently it is of paramount importance to maintain an objective and neutral position regarding the autopsy findings.

The realization that the autopsy findings must be rapidly reported, and that the report will be critically scrutinized, should guide the approach to police shooting deaths and deaths in police custody. As with any death having medicolegal interest, as much as possible should be learned of the incident itself prior to the autopsy. Under no circumstances should the autopsy begin without adequate information about the incident. Withholding this information because it is "secret," "classified," or "confidential" is unacceptable, and the pathologist should refuse to examine the body until the information is forthcoming. If at all possible, the medical examiner or coroner should respond to the scene.

Once the body is at the morgue, everything concerning the case is done on a priority ("stat") basis, and with strict attention to detail. To ensure accuracy and reduce the possibility of error, all tests and procedures are double-checked. If at all possible, a second pathologist should be recruited at the autopsy to help ensure that details are not overlooked. Photographs should be extensive and in duplicate, preferably by using two cameras. Also, it is important to photograph the autopsy procedure itself to help document any injuries, the pathway of the projectile, etc. Any evidence obtained from the body, such as bullets, should be photographed *in situ* and after removal along with its labeled containers.

The autopsy report should be detailed and readable. Pertinent negatives (e.g., no laceration of the knuckles or mouth, etc.) are particularly important and should not be forgotten. Once the report is typed and corrected by the pathologist, it should be given to another person (preferably another pathologist) to review for clarity and to check for obvious errors (e.g., a liver weight of 180 g in an adult male). After the protocol is finalized and signed, attach a neat body diagram that simply indicates the location of major injuries and/or the pathways of the projectiles.

We have found it extremely helpful to have a meeting about 24 hr after the incident. The meeting is attended by the medical examiner and/or coroner, the police investigators, crime laboratory personnel, and a prosecuting attorney. Each presents the results of his or her phase of the investigation. Further investigative efforts are then planned as a result of the shared information. Within three working days after the incident, the autopsy report and the entire case file are reviewed by the medical examiner along with others of the department involved with the case (toxicologist, forensic investigator, etc.). Another review is held 2 weeks after the incident to assure that everything has been satisfactorily completed.

MASS DISASTER

Successful management of a mass disaster requires a plan of action formulated well in advance of the incident. The plan should be carefully written in a step-by-step fashion and periodically reviewed with all members of the department. The plan of action eventually developed will, of course, depend on the type of community served and the anticipation as to what type of disaster is likely to occur. In a large metropolis, virtually anything is possible, but in smaller communities the potential for a mass disaster, and the possible varieties of mass disaster, become limited. Regardless of community size or the adequacy of the existing medical examiner facility, the following considerations are of paramount importance in formulating a mass disaster plan:

1. Define "mass disaster."
2. Anticipate the possible types of mass disaster in the community.
3. Have a list of questions for whoever notifies the medical examiner of a mass disaster.
4. Have a clearcut system of notification, complete with names and telephone numbers, for all who will be involved with the investigation or body handling.
5. Anticipate problems of body removal and storage.
6. Plan for additional telephone lines.
7. Plan for control of the concerned public and the news media (i.e., both physical and telephone security must be maintained).
8. Designate a person or mechanism to release information to citizens and the news media.
9. Enlist interagency cooperation and assign areas of jurisdiction.
10. Prepare a "disaster kit."
11. Ensure that all concerned have immediate access to the written disaster plan and an updated list of the telephone contact list.

A mass disaster is defined as single incident that generates a number of bodies that overwhelms your system or exceeds the storage facility. Thus, if your morgue has a capacity for 10 bodies, then 10 bodies from one incident would trigger the implementation of the disaster plan. However, you may choose to reduce this number if you are virtually the only pathologist available and have a very limited support staff.

Upon receiving notification of a mass disaster, obtain the following information:

1. The nature of the incident.
2. Estimated number of dead at the scene.
3. Estimated number transported to local hospitals.
4. Location of the scene.
5. Access to the scene (location of police command post).
6. Current status of rescue and investigative efforts.
7. When the medical examiner staff will be needed at the scene for investigative purposes and for body removal.
8. The presence of fire, dangerous chemicals, or nuclear radiation.
9. Who is in charge of the scene.
10. What agencies are or will be investigating the incident.

These questions are appropriate when the mass disaster is relatively localized, as in a hotel fire or commercial airline crash. Flash floods, earthquakes, civil insurrections (riots), etc. often preclude any scene investigation. In such circumstances, bodies will be delivered to the morgue from a variety of locations and quite possibly by a variety of personnel (police, ambulance, etc.), over a wide time range (hours to days or more).

When the scene is essentially an entire community, it becomes imperative that those who remove the bodies to the morgue do not remove wallets, purses, jewelry, clothing, etc., since these items will be crucial in attempts at identification. Also, it is critical that all the bodies from one site be transported together and not separated by sex, age, etc. This is important because the identification of one member of a group may easily lead to the identification of others in that group, particularly if it is a family unit.

From the perspective of a medical examiner, immediate scene response is not required, nor is it desired. Take advantage of the lead time: notify all who will be involved (dentists, body removal services, etc.), clear out the morgue (notify funeral homes, etc. to remove bodies), and get organized. Don't forget that routine cases will also be coming in along with the disaster victims, and these must also be anticipated.

Once a relatively localized mass disaster scene is safe (fire is put out, etc.) and secure, the medical examiner staff may proceed. The entire area should be photographed and sketched. Stakes with numbered flags or tags should be placed near each body and body part and adequately recorded. As each numbered body or body part is removed and placed in a body bag, an inventory is made of the clothing, jewelry, money, wallets, etc. These are also placed in the body bag for identification and so that the valuables may be returned to the next of kin. The purpose for the inventory at the scene is not only to prevent a mixup later on, but also to have a witnessed account as to what was actually present. Next of kin often claim that the deceased had certain jewelry or money on him or her and that it was stolen. Also, if these items are recorded at the scene, and the body arrives at the morgue without them, then one can be sure that theft indeed did occur. The scene inventory, therefore, helps prevent both fraud and theft. As the bodies are removed, be sure to keep a record of which bodies were close together; again, in a mass disaster, families and acquaintances often die together, and this aids greatly in identification.

As the bodies are brought to the morgue (or whatever facility is serving as a morgue, such as an airline hanger), they should be inprocessed and accessioned as usual. Efforts are then directed to each body to determine the cause and/or mechanism of death, and identification.

In an event such as an airplane crash, the cause of death is the same for all: "airplane crash" is simply put on the death certificate. Mechanisms of death, however, may vary: blunt force injury, drowning, inhalation of noxious fumes, etc. These mechanisms of death are identified by autopsy and toxicologic studies. In any event, one must make the decision as to whether all or only some of the bodies will be autopsied. This decision will, of course, be dictated by a multitude of practical factors. At the minimum, however, autopsies should be performed on all those for whom identification is a problem, and on those who may conceivably have been responsible for the disaster (e.g., the crew of an airplane).

The medical examiner facility will be deluged with telephone calls from concerned relatives and acquaintances and from the news media. To prevent chaos, plan for additional telephone lines and personnel (even volunteers). These personnel should attempt to have the relatives provide medical and dental records of the deceased, and describe any identifying scars, marks, tattoos, jewelry, clothing, etc. that may help in identification. Designate one person to provide news releases. One may consider establishing one telephone line exclusively for the news media. This may be handled by one person or by a recorded message with pertinent information, including when updates will be available.

Finally, in formulating a disaster plan, anticipate a worst possible scenario: mass burial. A provision should be made for one individual to have the authority to order a mass burial under certain circumstances. For example, a nuclear explosion resulting in extensive radioactive contamination of the bodies may preclude any type of adequate examination. For safety reasons, the only feasible course of action might be presumptive identification and mass burial in lead coffins.

In preparation for a mass disaster, prepare a "disaster kit." The kit should be tailored to anticipated problems, weather, terrain, and a host of other factors unique to your area.

REFERENCES

The following list of references is selected to provide the most practical information and help for the pathologist. The articles and books cited are chosen, in general, because they offer guidelines to both general and specific approaches, discuss specific techniques, or significantly expand upon chapters and subjects found in the general texts of medicolegal death investigation.

Selected References

General, Medicolegal Death Investigation

1. Moritz AR: Classical mistakes in forensic pathology. *Am J Clin Pathol* 26:1383–1397, 1956.
2. Spitz WU, Fisher RS: Medicolegal Investigation of Death—Guidelines for the Application of Pathology to Crime Investigation, ed 2. Springfield, Charles C Thomas, 1980.
3. Curran WJ, McGarry AL, Petty CS: Modern Legal Medicine, Psychiatry and Forensic Science. Philadelphia, F.A. Davis, 1980.
4. Wright RK, Wetli CV: A Guide to the forensic autopsy—conceptual aspects. In Sommers SC, Rosen PP (eds): *Pathology Annual,* Part 2, 16:273–288, 1981.
5. Adelson L: The Pathology of Homicide. Springfield, Charles C Thomas, 1974.

Crime Scene Investigation, Preserving Evidence

6. Fox RH, Cunningham CL: Crime Scene Search and Physical Evidence Handbook. U.S. Dept. of Justice, Law Enforcement Assistance Administration, National Institute of Law Enforcement and Criminal Justice, October 1973 (Superintendent of Documents, U.S. Government Printing Office, Washington, D.C., 20402).
7. Svensson A, Wendel O, Fisher BAJ: Techniques of Crime Scene Investigation, ed 3. New York, Elsevier, 1981.
8. Moenssens AA, Inbau FE: Scientific Evidence in Criminal Cases, ed 2. Mineola, New York, The Foundation Press, 1978.
9. Mittleman RE, Goldberg HS, Waksman DM: Preserving evidence in the emergency department. *Am J Nursing* 83:1652–1656, 1983.

Personal and Religious Objections to the Autopsy

10. Hirsch CS: Talking to the family after an autopsy. *Arch Pathol Lab Med* 108:513–514, 1984.
11. Autopsy in Jewish law and the Israeli autopsy controversy. In Rosen F: *Studies in Torah Judaism (Modern Medicine and Jewish Law)*. New York, Yeshiva University Department of Special Publication, 1972, pp. 132–154.

Firearms

12. DiMaio VJM: Gunshot Wounds. New York, Elsevier, 1985.
13. Brissie RM, Collum ES: Shotgun wounds, multiple probes and shielding effects as adjuncts to determining position of the deceased at time of injury. *J Forensic Sci* 25:528-532, 1980.

Sharp Force Injuries

14. Rao VJ, Hart R: Tool mark determination in cartilage of stabbing victim. *J Forensic Sci* 28:794–799, 1983.

Blunt Force Injuries

15. Contastavlos DL: Massive subarachnoid hemorrhage due to laceration of the vertebral artery associated with fracture of the transverse process of the atlas. *J Forensic Sci* 16:40–56, 1971.
16. Mittleman RE, Wetli CV: The threaded bolt injury pattern. *J Forensic Sci* 27:567–571, 1982.
17. Rao VJ: Patterned injury and its evidentiary value. *J Forensic Sci* 31:768–772, 1986.
18. Zugibe FT, Costello JT: Identification of the murder weapon by intricate patterned injury measurements. *J Forensic Sci* 31:771–773, 1986.

Motor Vehicle Injuries

19. Blackbourne D: Injury–vehicle correlations in the investigation of motor vehicle accidents. In Wecht CL (ed): *Legal Medicine Annual, 1980*. Philadelphia, W.B. Saunders, 1980.

20. Van Kirk DJ: A scientific approach to documenting evidence for accident reconstruction. *J Forensic Sci* 29:806–815, 1984.
21. Horowitz R, Siegel J, Flaster M, et al: Injury patterns in motor vehicle fatalities. *J Forensic Sci* 32:167–172, 1987.

Drowning and Diving Fatalities

22. Davis JH: Bodies found in water. *Am J Forensic Med Pathol* 7:291–297, 1986.
23. Findley T: An autopsy protocol for skin and scuba diving deaths. *Am J Clin Pathol* 67:440–443, 1977.
24. Marraccini JV, Friedman PL: Scuba death due to asthmatic bronchitis, air embolism and drowning. American Society of Clinical Pathologists Forensic Pathology Check Sample No FP86-6 (FP-149), 1986.

Mechanical Asphyxiation

25. Mittleman RE, Wetli CV: The fatal café-coronary. *JAMA* 247:1285–1288, 1982.
26. Mittleman RE: Fatal choking in infants and children. *Am J Forensic Med Pathol* 5:201–210, 1984.
27. Luke JL, Reay DT, Eisele JW, et al: Correlation of circumstances with pathological findings in asphyxial deaths by hanging: a prospective study of 61 cases from Seattle, WA. *J Forensic Sci* 30:1140–1143, 1985.
28. Perrot LJ, Froede RC, Jones AM: Asphyxiation by hanging in two young hispanic children—homicide, suicide or accidental death? A review of pediatric hangings. *Am J Forensic Med Pathol* 6:284–288, 1985.
29. Perper JA, Sobel MN: Identification of fingernail markings in manual strangulation. *Am J Forensic Med Pathol* 2:45–48, 1981.
30. Reay DT, Eisele JW: Death from law enforcement neck holds. *Am J Forensic Med Pathol* 3:253–258, 1982.
31. Koiwai EK: Death allegedly caused by the use of ''choke holds'' (shime-waza). *J Forensic Sci* 32:419–432, 1982.
32. Petty, CS: Topsy-turvy (positional asphyxia). American Society of Clinical Pathologists Forensic Pathology Check Sample No FP86–2 (FP–145). *Forensic Pathology* Vol 28, No 2, 1986.
33. Lowery S, Wetli CV: Sexual asphyxia—a neglected area of study. *Dev Behav* 4:19–39, 1982.
34. Hazelwood, RR, Dietz PE, Burgess AW: Autoerotic Fatalities. Lexington, MA, Lexington Books, D.C. Heath & Company, 1983.

Sexual Assault

35. Enos WF, Beyer JC: Spermatozoa in the anal canal and rectum and in the oral cavity of female rape victims. *J Forensic Sci* 23:231–233, 1978.
36. Enos WF, Beyer JC: The importance of examining skin and hair for semen in sexual assault cases. *J Forensic Sci* 26:605–607, 1981.
37. Deming JE, Mittleman RE, Wetli CV: Forensic science aspects of fatal sexual assault on women. *J Forensic Sci* 28:572–576, 1983.
38. Enos WF, Beyer JC: Examination of the rape victim. In Wiecking DK (ed):

Medico-Legal Bulletin Vol 33, No 3, May-June 1984. Virginia State Health Dept., Office of the Medical Examiner, 9 North 14th St., Richmond VA 23219.

Bitemarks

39. Mittleman RE, Stuver WC, Souviron R: Obtaining saliva samples from bitemark evidence. *FBI Law Enforcement Bulletin* 49:16–19, 1980.
40. Sperber ND: Bitemark evidence in crimes against persons. *FBI Law Enforcement Bulletin* 50:16–19, 1981.
41. Sopher IM: Bitemark analysis, American Society of Clinical Pathologists Forensic Pathology Check Sample No ST82–3 (ST–122), 1982.
42. Souviron R, Mittleman RE, Valor J: Obtaining the bitemark impression (mold) from skin. *FBI Law Enforcement Bulletin* 51:8–11, 1982.
43. Rao VJ, Souviron R: Dusting and lifting the bite print: a new technique. *J Forensic Sci* 19:326–330, 1984.

Fire and Arson

44. Kantrowitz SB: Expert testimony and scientific evidence in arson-related cases. *J Forensic Sci* 26:142–152, 1981.
45. Eckert WG: The medicolegal and forensic aspects of fires. *Am J Forensic Med Pathol* 2:347–357, 1981.
46. O'Connor JJ: Practical Fire and Arson Investigation. New York, Elsevier, 1987.

Electrical Deaths

47. Wright RK, Davis JH: The investigation of electrical deaths—a report of 220 fatalities. *J Forensic Sci* 25:514–521, 1980.
48. Dutra FR: Electrical burns of the skin. *Am J Forensic Med Pathol* 2:309–312, 1981.
49. Mitchell EK, Davis JH: Electrocution by street lighting. *J Forensic Sci* 29:836–842, 1984.
50. Liebler GE: Ground versus earth, there is a difference. *J Forensic Sci* 29:550–556, 1984.

Drug-Related Deaths

51. Baselt RC: Disposition of Toxic Drugs and Chemicals in Man, ed 2. Davis, CA, Biomedical Publication, 1982.
52. Wetli CV: Investigation of drug-related deaths—an overview. *Am J Forensic Med Pathol* 5:111–120, 1984.
53. Reay DT Eisele JW, Ward R, et al: A procedure for the investigation of anesthetic/surgical deaths. *J Forensic Sci* 30:822–827, 1985.
54. Wetli CV: Fatal cocaine intoxication—a review. *Am J Forensic Med Pathol* 8:1–9, 1987.

Fatal Child Abuse

55. Zumwalt RE, Hirsch CS; Subtle fatal child abuse. *Human Pathol* 11:167–174, 1980.

56. Mitchell EK, Davis JH: Spontaneous births into toilets. *J Forensic Sci* 29:591–596, 1984.
57. Davis JH, Rao VJ, Valdes-Dapena M: Forensic approach to the starved child. *J Forensic Sci* 29:663–669, 1984.
58. Kanda M, Thomas JN, Lloyd OW: The role of forensic evidence in child abuse and neglect. *Am J Forensic Med Pathol* 6:7–15, 1985.
59. Wagner GN: Crime scene investigation in child-abuse cases. *Am J Forensic Med Pathol* 7:94–99, 1986.
60. Mittleman RE, Mittleman HS, Wetli CV: Pattern injuries in child abuse. *Am J Nursing* 87:1185–1188, 1987.

Mass Disaster

61. McCormick MM: The National Transportation Safety Board and the investigation of civil aviation and transportation accidents. *Am J Forensic Med Pathol* 1:239–243, 1980.
62. Gilliland MCF, McDonough ET, Fossum RM, et al.: Disaster planning for air crashes—a Retrospective analysis of Delta Airlines flight 191. *Am J Forensic Med Pathol* 7:308–316, 1986.

Unidentified and Skeletal Remains

63. Fierro MF (ed): CAP Handbook for Postmortem Examination of Unidentified Remains. Skokie, IL, College of American Pathologists, 1986.
64. Brothwell DR: Digging Up Bones, ed 2. London, British Museum of Natural History, 1972.
65. Morse D, Duncan J, Stoutamire J (eds): Handbook of Forensic Archeology and Anthropology. Published by the editors, distributed by Bill's Bookstore, 107 South Copeland, Tallahassee, FL 32304.
66. Froede RC, Froede SM, Birnby WH: Systems for human identification. In Sommers SC, Rosen PP (eds) *Pathology Annual, 1981,* Part 1. New York, Appleton-Century-Crofts, 1981, pp. 337–365.

Index

F

G

H